Praise for *1
Addiction, Yoga, and Getting Well*

"A meaningful book on the role of spirituality in recovering from addiction and finding freedom. If you or anyone you love struggles to create that essential connection, this is a must-read."

— Elena Brower, best-selling author of *Practice You*

"Rolf provides accessible tools and reflective resources to support readers in staying curious, open, and calm. His decades of sobriety, study, and dedication are evident in every lesson of this book."

— Melody Moore, Ph.D., founder and Executive Director of Embody Love Movement Foundation

"Rolf Gates has broken new ground through the skillful, timely, and necessary integration of classical yoga philosophy, Buddhist meditation teachings, and the 12-step approach to overcoming addiction. This powerful trinity is a perfect salve for this exact moment in history."

— Tommy Rosen, founder of Recovery 2.0
and author of *RECOVERY 2.0*

"Combining heartfelt stories and insights with prompts for personal inquiry, Gates guides and supports the reader to navigate and transcend their own stories and limitations. Rolf's book is a gem that opens the realm of infinite possibilities through mindfulness, introspection, and application."

— Melanie Klein, empowerment coach, professor of Sociology and Women's Studies, and author of *Yoga Rising*

"Rolf Gates offers his whole self to those seeking healing and truth, providing a pathway to freedom through reflective self-inquiry, daily inspiration, and the practice of non-judgmental awareness. Using the wisdom traditions of yoga and Buddhism, Rolf elevates the field and offers tools that help so many others build capacity for self-regulation, resilience, and real happiness."

— David Lipsius, president and CEO of Yoga Alliance
and Yoga Alliance Foundation

Daily Reflections *on* Addiction, Yoga, *and* Getting Well

ALSO BY ROLF GATES

Meditations on Intention and Being

Meditations from the Mat

Daily Reflections

on Addiction, Yoga,

and Getting Well

ROLF GATES

HAY HOUSE, INC.
Carlsbad, California • New York City
London • Sydney • New Delhi

Published in the United States by: Hay House, Inc.: www.hayhouse.com® • *Published in Australia by:* Hay House Australia Pty. Ltd.: www.hayhouse.com.au • *Published in the United Kingdom by:* Hay House UK, Ltd.: www.hayhouse.co.uk • *Published in India by:* Hay House Publishers India: www.hayhouse.co.in

Cover design: Kathleen Lynch • *Interior design:* Joe Bernier

Cataloging-in-Publication Data is on file with the Library of Congress

Tradepaper ISBN: 978-1-4019-5396-6
e-book ISBN: 978-1-4019-5397-3

11 10 9 8 7 6 5 4 3
1st edition, September 2018

Printed in the United States of America

To Wendy and Jude

Contents

Introduction

Learning Separation

We are born innocent. There is no desire to find or to cause pain in some corner of our hopes and dreams. We make our first connections from a place of wonder. The smell of grass, the way the earth feels under our feet after a rain, the sound of snow whispering down through a nighttime sky—all are verses from the song in our hearts. Watching clouds pass through a summer sky, we are neither judging nor wishing things were different. Then we are taught to separate this from that, you from me. Before we know what has happened, we are labeling things and reacting to our labels. Penny is a cat, Max is a dog, Steve is a boy, you are a girl. The smells, the sounds, the breeze on our skin belong to a world we must find ourselves in. A blissful we becomes an anxious me.

I became an anxious me before my first memory. I have had to reflect, to put the pieces together, to understand what it was like to have an unfiltered experience. I have no memory of a time before the adults around me were filled with fear and anger. Life's beauty was something I glimpsed like the sky through prison bars. Our country was in a war of unimaginable ugliness. Our society had been driven mad by the belief that some people were "black" and others were "white," my parents were trapped in a life that didn't work, and as if these challenges weren't enough I had been adopted into an alien culture that was not sure I was really human. There was no peace, no belonging, no time when there would be.

I had a place where I could go to escape the overwhelming feelings that filled my days. When I watched television, I entered a world that welcomed me unconditionally. The characters I met there became the charming friends my heart ached for. The heroes offered a different sort of grown-up. These grown-ups lived without fear, often with great kindness. I found a home for myself in this world. I chose my relationship to TV over homework, friendship, family. There were consequences, but whatever "trouble" I found myself in faded into the background as I entered a world of laughter and adventure.

There is a scene in *Percy Jackson & the Olympians: The Lightning Thief*, one of my children's favorite movies, in which the heroes find themselves in the mythic land of the lotus-eaters. Our heroes are in Las Vegas. The casino they end up in is actually owned and operated by the lotus-eaters. For several days they dance and gamble in timeless bliss. One of them gets wise to the situation and alerts the others. As they wake up, they are faced with a dilemma: Is reality really better than an endless party? As a child, I did not have to spend any time on that one. On TV, there was always a place for me.

People like me find people like me. I sat in the back of the class with the other boys who had wounds they would never talk about or heal from. We did not listen, we did not cooperate, we did not care. In fourth grade during standardized testing, I got some questions wrong on purpose because I did not want to lose my identity. The wounded children were my tribe. Eventually they let me know they were smoking pot. One of my best friends started in sixth grade; I started in eighth. The first few times I got high, the experience was okay, but what I really loved was what the process gave me. From the start, getting high made me a part of something. I had found my way.

Learning Surrender

In *Percy Jackson*, the victims of the lotus-eaters live out their doom at an eternal party. In my version of the story, I had to live out my addiction in a Newtonian world of consequences. Life requires an abundance of wisdom and energy, and using robbed me of both. By the time I was 26 years old, I was several years past done. There had been coaches and teachers who had tried to help me with my wrestling or with my studies, but these had never been my problem. There is a saying that if you ask the wrong questions, you'll get the wrong answers. Until I found myself talking to an addictions counselor, I had never been asked the right questions. The counselor asked me if I would go to a 12-step meeting. It was the right question. I gave the right answer.

I was taken to my first meeting by a man who had survived four tours in Vietnam. He explained the nature of my illness and the experience of recovery. I was distracted by the emotional agony of dying an alcoholic death, but I got the point. I went to the meeting with him, brought home the book they gave me, and followed the instructions I found within its pages. The book's authors suggested that they were people like me. They said people like me need to pray for help. I tried it. It worked. On May 21, 1990, I prayed for help. I have not needed to drink since.

As the sober days began to add up, I learned that the change in my life was called surrender. I had stepped back and let go. Surrender creates a space for something new to enter your life. I was living in the presence of something new. It started as a good night's sleep. I was coming to my senses. Colors, sounds, tastes, even laughter was happening in a new way. Within just a couple of weeks, I began experiencing waves of empathetic joy for the people around me. I was deeply moved by their struggles, their courage, their victories. My heart began to speak to me very loudly. I cried a lot, tears that felt like waking up. The biggest change was the way the suffering of my active addiction had been replaced with a sense of communion with a divine energy that resonated through every aspect of my experience.

I had hard work to do. I went to rehab, I walked sober through the process of letting the world know I was an addict, I made amends. Much of my first year or two of sobriety was spent in dread of going back to drinking, but there was never a moment when I did not feel the presence of the divine. I was a wave that had forgotten the ocean. The act of surrender had allowed me to remember.

Learning Service

Nine months sober found me living in Boston with roommates, going to meetings every day, and "working a program." Working a program of recovery meant that I was applying the spiritual disciplines suggested at 12-step meetings. The people at the meetings combined humility with courage in a way that felt utterly compelling. The ones who inspired me the most had found a way to dedicate their new sober life to the betterment of others. When I heard someone speak of this in a meeting, I knew I was listening to the reason for my existence. The difficulties of active addiction, the challenges of active recovery, the losses, the sorrows, the uncertainty, the disappointments, the humanity—all had prepared me to be of service.

From the start I did what I could. I made coffee at meetings. I helped newcomers get to meetings. I went to sober parties, weddings, funerals. Most of all I tried to treat those around me with the kindness I was learning in meetings. As the days turned into years, I learned that the combination of "working a program" and helping others created a self-sustaining dynamic in my life. Serving others reminded me of the beauty of a sober life, and living sober inspired me to serve others.

Learning Stillness

Once you put the drink down, you have to deal with the person who drank in the first place. In my case, what was left after the drinking was someone whose life had been defined by trauma the way a glass defines the shape of the water it holds. Recovery from addiction is a redefinition. The story of addiction becomes a story of recovery. The story of loss becomes a story of forgiveness. The story of trauma becomes a story of resilience. This transformation unfolds across the landscape of our relationships.

I joined a community, I found friendship, I learned to work for others, I learned to work with others, I found love, I made my peace with life on life's terms. I was able to accomplish all of this without actually befriending myself. The human will is strong. I wanted to heal, and I did it the only way I knew how. When I needed to deal with myself, I found a distraction, a desire, an aversion, a delusion. I had never sat with myself or spent any time feeling what it was like to be me here now. I did not know how that would help.

As I healed, the intimacy of my relationships intensified. My friendships in early recovery had a tumultuous quality. It seemed everyone wanted the best for one another but had no idea how to make that happen. I had what amounted to zero sense of how I was showing up in relationships. This was exacerbated by the fact that I could not see or feel the intensity of the expectations I was putting on the people in my life. In spite of myself, I made progress in my career and found someone who would marry me. This only intensified the requirement that I develop the capacity to deal with my inner life while staying true to the commitments I had made in my outer life. It was a capacity I had no ability to cultivate without significant guidance and support. The final nail in my coffin of suffering was the fact that there was not even a word, let alone a language, in my world for what I needed next. All I could do was feel the pain of lack.

If a colleague, a friend, a client, or my partner behaved in a way that I found difficult, I would react. Twelve-step work had given me some valuable resources in those situations, including the ability to be clear about my intention, the desire to live non-violently, and the commitment to take responsibility for my part, but I faced these situations without the ability to live skillfully in my own body, my own heart, my own mind. I sought out yoga and meditation without any hope that I would be able to use them to gain the skill I lacked. All I wanted was relief. I wanted a place to go where I could drop the weight off my shoulders for a while. Where I could feel safe. Where I could remember the love with which the divine held me. What I found was a group of people who had been like me and had found a solution.

For the second time in my life I had come up against a problem I could not solve, only to stumble into a room where people were solving it. The meetings where I learned to live sober had been held in humble and gritty rooms, places where the grandiosity of the addict is abandoned in favor of connection with other human beings. The classrooms where I learned to be still in the presence of love smelled great, had soft lighting, and possessed a palpable presence of the sacred. The chaos of an unexamined inner life was abandoned in favor of a life of self-awareness within the sanctuary of my own loving-kindness. It is a magnificent invitation to meet myself on sacred ground among those who are dedicated to the purity of their heart's intention. This is what I found when I needed it most.

I am writing this book a quarter century later, looking back on the way yoga and meditation have made possible the life my young, sober self yearned for. It is my hope that all those who are recovering from the disease of addiction will find what I have found in these practices. It is my hope that this book will be a support to you as you make it so.

Learning to Remember

It is said that a teacher reminds the student until she remembers. The daily reflections format offers us a chance to glance at a line or two before we head out into our day. The idea is that we are already committed to a path of recovery but may need a little support remembering what that means. I organized these reminders following the Buddha's instructions that the path to freedom possesses a basic logic.

On the path to freedom, we will need to remember:

> View: The nature of addiction, recovery, and living free
>
> Intention: The willingness to go to any length to live our recovery one day at a time
>
> Truth: The cultivation of an honest effort in service of an honest life
>
> Action: Non-violence in thought, word, and deed
>
> Service: Giving it away to keep it
>
> Effort: Finding the middle between doing and being one breath at a time
>
> Mindfulness: Choosing to be present without attachment one breath at a time
>
> Concentration: To be of one mind—one heart— one purpose

These reminders form a path that is a circle. We can enter it at any point. We can choose any direction upon it. The destination will always be home.

Learning to See

For the past couple of years I have been teaching at Spirit Rock Meditation Center, where I have been a student for many years. It is a way to give back to a community that has given me so much. During a recent spring retreat, I got to have series of breakfasts with Bhante Buddharakkhita, Uganda's first Buddhist monk. For a few quiet mornings, I had this superb teacher to myself. He began his teachings by reminding me that a human being is a verb, not a noun.

We are a process

Life is a process

This book is a process

The purpose of this book is to help. It travels down the Buddha's eightfold way to the end of suffering. The wisdom it reflects comes from the Yoga Sutras, 12-step programs, and from the Buddha himself. These three perspectives on finding freedom combine the way instruments or voices combine to create a melody.

Whenever you find yourself listening to this melody, remember that you are a verb, not a noun. You are a process that has called forth this teaching for this day. This teaching will not be new to you; rather, it will be reminding you of what you already know. Reminding you of who you already are.

May it find you safe
May it find you healthy
May it find you happy
May it find you free

Namaste,
Rolf

Chapter One

The View

A World War I veteran named Bill Wilson gained a series of insights into the nature of addiction. He saw how to understand the problem, how to get well, how to stay well, how to help others. Bill W. created a group process around these insights that became the modern 12-step movement. This process has made possible the adoption of sobriety by millions of addicts around the world. The impact of Bill Wilson's life on countless other lives demonstrates the power of seeing our way to freedom. The Buddha gave this power a name: wise view. To have the view is to know the cause of suffering, to know the way to freedom, and to possess the will for the journey. Our first chapter will examine the view.

1.

A friend of mine who would one day die of his addiction was living on Maine's coastline attending a two-year program at a prestigious photography institute. I would travel north from Boston to visit him, spending a few days in a life that made more sense to me than my own. One weekend I arrived early. My friend would not be available until the evening. I picked up some wine and went to a spot on the coast. For a number of hours, I sat at the edge of a forest looking upon the vastness of the Atlantic Ocean. As the wine kicked in, I felt a deep peace settle over me. My mind grew still, my body softened, my heart opened. I felt connected to the timeless, eternal now. At a cookout later that night, I would be embarrassingly drunk, but the moment at the water's edge has stayed with me.

Carl Jung expressed his bewilderment at the difficulty of treating addiction. He theorized that the illness was spiritual in nature. He thought the person in question might recover if she experienced a spiritual transformation. To understand addiction, we must reflect on what the addict is seeking.

Reflection

What were you seeking in active addiction? What are you seeking now? Make a list.

2.

My teacher Bhante began his teachings by telling me that the human is a verb. She is a process. Her body is a process. Her feelings, perceptions, mental states, and consciousness are a process. To listen to the sound of a bell is to observe a process arising, changing, vanishing. A school year, a childhood, a career, an experience of well-being, an experience of suffering—all arise, change, vanish. This much we understand. But through what Einstein called an optical illusion of consciousness, we think of ourselves as a singular intellectual artifact. We think we are a noun. The research on the subject tells us that for survival, we retain the memory of negative experiences far more readily than our positive ones. So not only are we a noun. We are a noun whose experience skews to the negative.

The addict has less tolerance for this state than others. Why the addict finds her experience of living as a negative noun unmanageable is moot. She does, and she seeks relief in active addiction. The Buddha sought relief as well. The difference is that his path led to liberation. The addict's way leads to suffering. We are all on a path to somewhere; wise view is knowing where it leads.

Reflection

When has your path led you to happiness? What adds up to a good day?

3.

On our second morning together, I asked Bhante to explain the difference between ignorance and delusion. He said ignorance is like being blind. In ignorance, we cannot see at all. In delusion, we think that something that will make us unhappy will make us happy. In delusion, we see backward. This offers us an important starting point. Have you ever thought something would make you happy only to have it cause unhappiness? Have you ever shook your head and wondered what you were thinking? What was your mental state? What was your emotional state? How did you feel when you were seeing backward?

Reflection

Describe a time when you wanted something that made you unhappy. Describe the thoughts, emotions, mental states, circumstances. Reflect for a while on the mental state of delusion.

4.

On the third day, I asked Bhante to explain the concept of skillful and unskillful mental states. That morning in meditation, I had discovered the ability to rest in a "skillful mental state," which is to say I found myself resting in a spacious connection to the present moment. The contracted states of wanting, not wanting, and delusion were not present. I could feel when they would begin to arise. My mind would start moving. My body would begin to tense. Then I would rest back into connection. My mind would become still while my body relaxed. I was fascinated by the ability to see *how* I was seeing. Could this be an important step in my process?

Bhante said that greed, hatred, and delusion were the three unskillful mind states. He went on to say that when greed or hatred arises, delusion follows. Craving anything distorts our view. The very intensity with which we want something to be, or not to be, distorts our ability to understand it. What a predicament the addict is in. Suffering intensely, the addict craves relief. Desperate for relief, the addict sees backward. Seeking happiness, the addict takes the path to unhappiness.

Reflection

Unpack a specific situation when wanting something or not wanting something made you a little (or a lot) nuts. Reflect on how craving sets us up for seeing backward.

5.

The Yoga Sutras describe the way the mind habitually turns away from the present moment, how this sets into motion the creation of a mind-made self that carves the world up into what it wants and what it does not want. In meditation we can observe this process unfold. Bhante says that watching is enough. Watching stabilizes the mind. As the mind stabilizes, the self falls away. Initially this falling away of the self is temporary, but over time we fall out of love with the self and into love with the present. The unskillful states of mind that cause us to see backward have only a tenuous hold on us if we can learn to reflect on them as opposed to reacting to them.

Attending 12-step meetings is the first way I learned to reflect on unskillful states of mind as opposed to reacting to them. As people spoke, I was able to see how an unskillful state of mind can arise, how it has an agenda separate from our well-being. Anger seeks revenge. Desire seeks fulfillment. Delusion thinks the drink that made us unhappy can make us happy again. Listening to people's stories unfold, I saw how my own mind worked when it contracted into craving, when it became attached to an outcome, and how these states of mind saw only what they wanted to see. Sitting in meetings, I learned to watch the mind.

Reflection

Reflect on how easy it is to see someone else caught up in an unskillful state of mind but how difficult it is to see when you are in it. What helps you gain perspective when you are caught in an unskillful state of mind? List a few aids: friends, enough rest, healthy eating, etc.

6.

There was a moment in rehab when I understood what the term "romancing the drink" meant. I had been doing it since middle school without realizing it. Sitting in French class, I would be thinking about the keg party on the weekend, or the pot I was going to buy later that day. I would work myself up into a state of desire that could not be reasoned with. Any warning lights, any twinges of common sense or self-preservation, would be steamrollered by the momentum of my attachment to getting what I wanted. Romancing the drink was the unskillful mind state that preceded the unskillful act of getting drunk. The mind state preceded the behavior.

Sitting in rehab, I saw the relationship between the mind state and the behavior. I saw that if I did not want the behavior, I could not afford to entertain the mind state. In that moment, I let go of romancing the drink. For many years, the anticipation of drinking sometime soon had comforted me. As I walked through the cold night at the U.S. Army Ranger School, I would think of buying a case of beer and showing up at my friend's house. As I sat through endless hours of schooling that held no charm for me, I would think of the release of "getting high" later. Romancing the drink had provided me with relief from situations I wanted to escape. This mental state had been a friend, but it could not accompany me into recovery any more than the actual substances I had abused over the years.

Reflection

Describe how you have romanced self-destructive behavior. How has this mental behavior been better than feeling what you were feeling? What has been the cost?

7.

Sitting in rehab, I saw the relationship between the mind state and the behavior that followed. I felt what meditation teachers call "the ouch of it." I felt how romancing the drink would lead to my doom. I felt the ouch of being caught in a river heading over the falls. I saw how this river had only one destination. I felt how powerless I was once I entered the river. I knew that if I wanted to live, I could not so much as dip my toe into the rushing river called romancing the drink.

The first Noble Truth of Buddhism states that we have the mental habit of choosing the path to suffering. The second Noble Truth says that we choose the path to suffering because we are in the habit of getting caught in unskillful mind states. The third Noble Truth states that we can abandon that habit. Sitting in rehab, I experienced this directly. I saw the habit. I felt into the pain it had caused and would surely cause again. I abandoned the habit.

Reflection

Reflect on why letting ourselves feel the ouch of a pattern is so important. How does this change our relationship to it? Going to meetings helped me feel the ouch of being lost in addiction. Meditating helped me feel into the mind states that led to addiction. My yoga mat is where I feel the bliss of letting go. What helps you feel?

8.

In meetings, I learned that "thinking the drink through" was the opposite of romancing the drink. It is the mental habit of evaluating a behavior to get clear about its logical consequences. If I do this, what usually happens? What are the logical consequences of this behavior on myself, my family, my friends, my colleagues at work, my community? What will be the effect of this choice? What do I already know about this behavior?

Thinking the drink through is associated with the left side of our prefrontal cortex. Researchers have determined that this part of the brain measurably thickens when someone meditates. The most profound evidence of this was observed while a monk practiced loving-kindness meditation in an MRI. Watching helps, but watching with kindness helps more. Sitting in meetings, I watched people I had grown to love think the drink through. It helped.

Reflection

For many of us, self-observation without judgment feels almost impossible to pull off. A 12-step meeting provides us a chance to practice with others before we are ready to turn a kind gaze toward our own behavior and inner life. Reflect on a person who has held you in a kind gaze. How has this made a difference in your life? When have you held others in a kind gaze? Why did you look at them this way? Can you imagine looking at yourself this way?

9.

The path to freedom begins with the ability to see with kindness. In meetings, you learn to listen with kindness. On a meditation cushion, you learn to watch with kindness. On a yoga mat, you learn to feel with kindness. If I do this, it feels like this. When my mind is focused, I am strong. When my mind wanders, I grow weak. The medium for understanding on a yoga mat is sensation. You learn to think the drink through by how things feel. How does it feel when I am attempting to pose as a noun? As a verb? How does it feel when I am in this body, this breath, this moment? What works? Can I feel into what works without judgment? Can I learn to learn with kindness? How does it feel when I am being kind?

Reflection

How does being kind change the way you are listening, seeing, feeling?

10.

Kindness is like placing our hand in a forest pool to touch the smooth surface of a stone on the bottom. Without kindness, we can see the stone but we cannot feel it. In a spiritual practice, the stone at the bottom of the pool is our heart. Today I draw a great deal of comfort from the fact that I kept coming back to my practice until I was willing to reach down through the water to feel the smooth surface of my heart.

Reflection

We are a verb. We are a process. Sometimes this process is guided by kindness. Sometimes it is guided by craving. Notice how you can feel the difference.

11.

When I first stepped onto a yoga mat, being kind to myself as a way to help myself learn had never occurred to me. The work I was doing with young people was about holding them with unconditional love. The tasks, the structure, the moments in our days together were a means to that end. I knew what others needed, but I could not translate that understanding into how to be with myself.

At meetings we say, "Let us love you until you can learn to love yourself." This was more than I could deal with. I accepted the help, the guidance, but knew nothing of letting someone love me. It had not been necessary. But as I rested in safety at the end of a yoga class, I knew that without love, addiction had been necessary. How do you let love in? Resting at the end of class, I could not let love in, but I could let the moment in. I could let the sweetness of the light from an evening sky in. I could let the firmness of the floor beneath me in. I could let the silence in, the stillness in. It was a beginning.

Reflection

Twelve-step meetings, meditation classes, and yoga classes are places where we learn to receive life's sweetness. As an addict, this part of our lives is often broken. How are you making a beginning?

12.

It is important to remember that if we are not careful, we will see things backward. Hoping to get, we will grasp with a closed hand, a closed mind, a closed heart. Hoping to give, we will forget to let go. If we are not careful, we will create the opposite of what we seek. The active addict has perfected this. The recovering addict is unlearning this. Our three practices (12-step, meditation, and yoga) can help us because they are able to meet us where we are. They have the ability to start with our closed fist, closed mind, and closed heart. We simply need to be willing to show up. One asks us to listen, another to watch, another to feel; nothing else—just, listening, watching, feeling. Slowly letting love in. Slowly letting life in.

I was in a yoga class one day, and the teacher told us to move from thinking to feeling. So I did. There it was. It had been there all along. Life.

Reflection

How are you letting life back in?

13.

If letting life back in is the solution, what is the problem? Yoga would say that we have the mental habit of turning away from life. Buddhism uses the word *contracting* instead of *turning away*. In either case, we mentally pull back from life. In 12-step programs, they say that the effort to manage life instead of living it has made life unmanageable. In all three cases, the problem isn't what we were addicted to. The problem is why we were using in the first place. We were using in an effort to control life instead of living life on life's terms. This effort places us on the road to suffering.

Reflection

This is a critical thing to know about ourselves. What is your relationship to control?

14.

There was an African American addict who lived in the Jim Crow South. When it was time for him to get sober, he was not allowed in the meetings in his hometown. Undeterred, he sat outside the meetings to listen to the teachings. This was enough. He held trainings for other African Americans so that they could bring what he had learned to others. Several decades later, a white woman asked him to teach her how to treat addicts. He did. She went on to found one of the first, if not the first, eating disorder clinics in the United States.

When I met her, she was in her 80s. Her center is called Shades of Hope, and if you spend time there, you are taught to understand addiction as an effort to manage the unmanageable. The addict wants to control how she feels, hoping that the predictable nature of her substance will make life predictable. *Control* is the key word. Our practices teach us to abandon control in favor of connection.

Reflection

Reflect on how much the desire for a specific experience has factored into your addiction. How has your addiction been about control? How has the desire for control made your life unmanageable?

15.

At a meditation retreat, the students often receive the same answer to any number of questions—questions about physical, emotional, or mental discomfort; sleepiness; anxiety; regret; insight. Whatever it is, they are instructed to "include it." I first heard this instruction during the early days of a retreat while detoxing from my caffeinated modern life. Through the fog I saw a teacher making a glib comment to someone in pain. The days passed, and the instruction to "include it" kept coming. With little else to do, I started trying to include things. As a pain would arise, my instinct was to try to escape or control the experience; instead I began softening to include the discomfort. I would not leave the breath or my connection to the present but would now bring a new phenomenon into the gentle gaze of mindfulness.

Including something is the opposite of coercing or fleeing it. The choice to include an experience is the opposite of the choice to control an experience. The addict who is learning to include more and more of her experience is learning a behavior far more effective than control. To include is to invite some new aspect of yourself to sit down, feel safe, and tell you her story.

Reflection

Begin to notice when you are having an internal reaction that you habitually flee or coerce, like a jealousy or an irritation you feel you are not supposed to have. Set aside a moment or two to include it, to be still and relaxed as you let yourself feel what it is like to be jealous or irritated or afraid—what it is like to be human.

16.

At meetings you are taught to include new experiences by learning to "identify, not compare." The defensiveness that shows up on a meditation cushion as the desire to coerce or abandon an experience shows up in a meeting as an attack on the messenger. "I was never that bad." "I can't relate to his story because I never went to prison." "I never did drugs. I only smoked pot." "I still had my job." "She never lost anything—what does she know about my life?" Take a breath, then include it.

Listen for how another's feelings were like your feelings—the fear, anger, sadness. When I listen, really listen, I hear myself. When I am awake, I find myself saying that I am like that too.

Reflection

Reflect on how judging or comparing makes you more alone. Reflect on how seeing yourself in someone else makes you less alone. Feel into the difference between control and connection.

17.

My children see much more than I do. They notice colors, patterns, changes in their environment, the way someone walks, the way people's faces reflect their emotions, the way the world is a verb. They understand this far better than I do. My mind grasps at an objective, a goal. Theirs are open to whatever the moment brings. I see what confirms the things I already believe. They see what there is to be seen. Noticing the difference is enough to begin a practice.

What happens to us? Why do children see more than their parents? What can adults do to regain their ability to see?

Reflection

How often does "getting somewhere" become an obstacle to being here?

18.

One of the challenges I face as a teacher is that my students are trying to get somewhere in a practice dedicated to being here. This leaning into the next moment is no small matter. It is a mental, physical, emotional, and energetic toll that competes with the precious, difficult work we do together. Part of the problem is that the goal has been described in terms that make it seem nearly unattainable. It tends to be a noun like *enlightenment* or *realization*, when the actual experience is a process. We are present, then we are present, then we are present, then we are present again—each moment of presence the same but different from the last. To make matters worse, this noun-goal that does not in any way resemble our verb-experience exists sometime in the future. By definition, it is not included in our present experience. If the good is "over there, sometime in the future," why not lean forward? Why not push, strive, grasp, or crave?

Why you do something is as important is how you do something. Supplying a "why" for my students' efforts that does not produce more suffering has not been as easy as it might seem. I have had to look very closely at my own experience. What works? Well, when I sit in the morning, eat a healthy breakfast, then give myself to wholesome tasks, my inner life slows enough for me to make better choices. It's like a batter being able to slow down the pitch. My practice slows things down so I can know what things taste like, smell like, *feel* like. My practice is the process of slowing things down in the service of making better choices.

Reflection

What helps you slow things down? What speeds things up? How can you tell?

19.

A person in 12-step recovery calls the set of disciplines she is employing to stay sober her program. A yoga person calls the set of disciplines she is using to make her life work her *sadhana*. The Buddhist follows a set of disciplines called the Buddha Dharma. The behavior is the same; the names are different. The individual employs a set of disciplines to make her life better. Define *better*? Along what path does our life unfold? The path our choices lay before us. To have a program, to have a *sadhana*, to follow the Buddha Dharma, is to live in hopes that skillful choice-making will set us on the path to freedom.

Our aim is to live in the space before a choice is made with intelligence, with heart. Our practice is dedicated to this aim. It stretches the moments we live in. So that a breath becomes long enough, so that a sensation can be eloquent, a heart can whisper, a mind can know, or a choice can express a simple prayer. On earth as it is in heaven.

Reflection

Reflect on the moment before you make a choice. What signals from the body, the breath, the emotions say stop, and which say go? What helps you to recognize the signals?

Buddha's Path to Freedom

The Buddha laid out three stages on the path to freedom. The first is the quest for gratification. In the second stage we begin to examine the price of gratification. In the third stage we seek freedom. The next few essays will be dedicated to this perspective on addiction.

20.

The first stage of Buddha's path to freedom should look familiar to anyone who has lived with addiction. The quest for gratification has an almost impenetrable logic: experiencing X is very gratifying so you want that experience. Young children experiencing dessert, adolescents experiencing sex, young adults experiencing success, finding love, gaining financial freedom are being introduced to the joys of gratification. The pure rush of gratification sets us on a quest that will be all many humans will ever know of life.

We think that if we get enough of what we want, we'll be happy. The fact that this has not been true does not matter because soon we will get what we want the way we want it. This perfect state will be a moment of redemption that will make up for all of the dead ends along the way. And in that moment, all the ways that the quest for gratification have failed us will be forgiven.

My redemption fantasy was the moment my hand would be raised for a gold medal in Olympic wrestling. I drank, I smoked pot, I had sex, but mostly I wanted respect. I wanted to be of value. Winning a gold medal at the Olympics would prove once and for all that I was worth the air that I breathed. I lay awake at night picturing that moment, the hand raised, feeling the gravity of what it would mean. Redemption.

Reflection

What are some of the stories you have told yourself about getting what you wanted? What has the pursuit of gratification been like?

21.

The quest for gratification is so compelling to us that we need to run out of road before we can stop. The wheels have to come off in some life-threatening way. We get cancer, someone close to us dies or leaves, our business fails, our marriage implodes. Addicts tend to bottom out after not one but a series of these types of experiences. Many addicts don't live that long, but some do. The survivors will question the quest for gratification. They wouldn't put it in those terms; they just know that they are sick and tired of being sick and tired.

Bill Wilson described this state as "incomprehensible demoralization." Simultaneously numb and in agony, we have no idea what to do. Caught up in the darkness, my sister's last words before she died from addiction were "I don't know what to do; I don't know what to do." The following morning, when I brought my mother the news, she cried, "It never stops; it never stops." We don't know when we started being this way. We don't know what to do now that we are this way. The only thing we know for sure is that we are caught like an animal in a trap. Then someone comes by with a key.

Reflection

How many times did the wheels come off before you were willing to try something new? What made you question the quest for gratification?

22.

The addict pays a high price to get to the second stage of Buddha's path to freedom. The toll of her addiction can be felt in every aspect of her life. Her body has been betrayed. Her heart, her mind, her loves, her passions, her friends, her family, her community, her dignity, her place in society—anything, everything that she has known or experienced has been sacrificed for another moment of gratification. This process has left her without the ability to respect or trust herself. At this stage, Bill Wilson said, "our bankruptcy as a going concern is completed."

Being broken helps. The next part of this process requires us to follow instructions closely. Someone comes by with a key. Staring up at her from our prison floor, we can't quite believe she is there or that it matters, but when she puts out her hand, we take it.

Reflection

How has being beaten down by addiction helped you to pay attention when someone is trying to help you?

23.

I met my first spiritual teacher at my second 12-step meeting. His name was Henry. He cared for me at the lowest point of my life. He taught me that I had value by valuing me. He picked me up, brought me to meetings, spent time with me afterward. He smiled when he saw me. He let me spend time at his house with his family. I have a scar from his puppy's sharp tooth that might as well have been put there by God in terms of what it means to me. Henry taught me to make my bed. He told me to consider how little time it takes to make your bed in the morning. He asked me to reflect on how it feels at the end of a long hard day to come home to a clean, well-made bed. He taught me to take care of myself because I was worth it. In the warmth of Henry's smile, I took my first steps on the path to freedom.

Reflection

What was it like for you when someone came by with a key?

24.

My heart thawed slowly. Much of early recovery was like finding the bodies trapped in the snow after an avalanche. Frozen in their last moments—new boots, worn parkas, bits of scarf. My sadness was overwhelming. My 12-step sponsor, Henry, knew this about me. He was kind to my sorrow. There were no answers for what broke my heart. There was no getting any of it back. I walked through the end of a life in a young body.

After a month or two, I discovered a new kind of laughter. It was a mixture of relief, joy, and togetherness that was the closest to happiness I had ever experienced. Henry had a few key phrases to trigger this sort of laughter. One of my favorites was Henry saying "what it was like" in his southern drawl. He would say the phrase, and then I would copy his drawl in an awful Boston way. We were referring to the suggestion that 12-step people reflect on what it was like to be stuck in the quest for gratification. Henry would look at some broken part of my life, lift an eyebrow, and drawl "what it was like." We would laugh until tears came to our eyes at what it was like and would be no more.

Reflection

Life has put people in your life who have not been afraid of your sadness. Thank them in your heart. Maybe thank them in person. Who has helped you laugh the laugh of freedom?

25.

In the second stage of Buddha's quest for freedom, we come to question the quest for gratification. The meditators just sit and watch it play out behind closed eyes. They don't have to go anywhere. It comes to them. The thoughts, the feelings, the hopes, the fears, the quest for gratification comes to them. A 12-step meeting works like a potluck. Everyone brings a little bit of wisdom: she's learned this, he's learned that. Together they create a teaching that has never been before. It is the teaching the group needs that night. The next day there will be a new one. As long as there are addicts learning to question the quest for gratification, they will never run out.

They say that by the time we have seen the light of a star, it has been dead for untold ages. We are seeing what has been. The wisdom of the second stage is like that, only instead of seeing the light of long-gone stars we are feeling the pain of long-gone actions. Sitting quietly, doing nothing, the meditator sits in the echo of past actions. Sitting quietly, sharing honestly, the 12-step group feels the pain of an ancient quest. Using the light cast by ancient worlds, the navigator charts a course to a new one.

Reflection

Does getting what you want make you happy? What is your experience? If not, what does make you happy?

26.

One Saturday morning I heard a young dancer talk about the day she took a drunken fall from a fire escape. There she was—young, intelligent, broken. It is the kind of story that stays with you because it speaks to a very large truth. No one ever outsmarts the disease of addiction. We have three options. Don't have it, die from it, or learn to live with it one day at a time. We learn to live with it the way we would learn to live with any other predator. When does it hunt? How does it hunt? What do you do when you meet one alone in the forest?

A student told me about observing grizzlies in Alaska with her son. She was on a tour and the guides told them to stay close to one another. The guide said the bears won't attack as long as you are in a group. Observing the quest for gratification is a lot like standing on a riverbank as grizzlies feed on salmon, armed only with a camera. Don't do it alone.

Reflection

What is it like when you are doing your spiritual work in the context of a spiritual community? What is it like when you try to do it alone?

27.

There are signs that things are getting better. There are signs that we are waking up. One is laughter. Another is tears. Compassion begins to replace fear or hatred. We become filled with a desire to help others. For me, two things happened almost simultaneously. I began to be aware of the presence some people call God. As this presence began to fill my days, I felt that I could no longer participate in violence against another human being. I was 26 when this happened. I was a military officer whose specialty was missions that entailed a high degree of violence, but there was no conflict in my heart. Violence had once been consistent with my sense of duty to my community. It was no longer. Being kind was now my duty.

In class, we talked about the moment when you are no longer living for what you can get and begin living for what you can give. As I made the shift from chasing gratification to questioning it, I had to reenvision my life's purpose. The question became "What am I here to give?"

Reflection

What are you here to give?

28.

We have created circles around the quest for gratification. When we begin to leave the chase, we have to find new circles. These circles support us as we examine the suffering caused by the chase. These circles support us as we discover a new purpose. The Buddhists describe this as finding refuge. We find refuge from our old belief system. We find refuge from a world that does not understand the change in our life. We find refuge for this new way of seeing. We find refuge for this new purpose. Together we create sacred ground. This ground will be beneath our feet, its dust a gentle presence. We will breathe in its scent as we take our first steps on the path to freedom.

Reflection

Describe a step you have taken from your circle out into the world.

29.

We are learning to love something. The cool in the morning, the smell of the earth after a rain, the random pace at which a 12-step meeting fills, the excited murmur in a yoga room before class starts, the way the heat from the sun is different from the heat of a fire, how birds sound like water moving across a streambed, the indescribable sincerity of a dog's love, the goodness in your own heart. We are learning to love life. The chase declares that life has not given us enough. In the quiet, as the chase begins to subside, we see the beauty of what life has given.

Reflection

What is something you are learning to love about your world?

30.

There is a special kind of choice we make when our heart is touched. It is not a result of careful calculation; it is not really a choice at all. It is an answer. Our heart calls. We respond. The step from considering the price of gratification to choosing the path to freedom is like this. We see the beauty of the path. Our heart opens. Our feet move. In the second stage, the path to freedom is revealed. In the third stage, we go where it leads.

For many of us, the path to freedom is revealed when we are trying to help someone else. We see her pain, her vulnerability. We feel how close her addiction has brought her to death. We feel the presence of beautiful possibility. We stand with her at the crossroads. The darkness is revealed. But look over there; can you see the light?

Reflection

Describe a moment when helping someone helped you to see more clearly.

31.

The ancient teacher Lao-Tzu wrote that when the wise hear the truth, they immediately embody it. For the rest of us, it is a process. Learning is a verb. The truth comes to us like so many grains of sand on the scales of our heart. It slowly gathers; then one day we are ready. We know it is the truth because it leads to freedom. We know we are ready because of the gladness in our hearts. When a bird takes flight, she is embodying the truth. When a caterpillar becomes a butterfly, she is embodying the truth. When we look into another's eyes with love, we are experiencing the truth. The movement from the question to the answer is a step toward the truth.

I was not sure what was happening during my first yoga class. It came, I flailed, it ended. Walking from that class to breakfast, there was a joy in my body that would never leave. I had learned where to go to find the truth in my cells. At a meeting during my first year of sobriety, I listened to a gentleman tell his story and felt a joy in my heart that would never leave. I had learned where to go to find the truth in my heart. When we find the truth, we stop looking and start living.

Reflection

What has the process of finding your truth about addiction been like? What is it like to seek but not find? What is it like to find?

32.

When I first started going to meetings, I was told that all I had to change was everything. We may have used anger, striving, proving, blaming, justification, and rationalization effectively on the quest for gratification, but we will find these of little use once we are living sober. The path to freedom requires a new skill set. These skills have a paradoxical bent to them. We learn to "give it away to keep it," to "turn the other cheek," to "surrender to win." The idea of "letting go" gets a lot of positive press as well, although no one ever tells us what to let go of or how. Not only are we walking a new path to a new future, but we must learn to walk all over again.

It is not a simple matter to change your life at any point. Many of us are in the midst of a great deal when we are asked to drop everything and start swimming for shore. I took several giant strides back in order to create the space I needed to learn what I had to learn. At 25 I was a highly paid professional in my chosen field. At 30 I was a waiter working lunches in hopes of someday getting the better-paid dinner shift. I had gone back to school full-time in a way that the world could not see or acknowledge. This might be our first great task on the path to freedom: to utterly abandon the way the world has taught us to evaluate ourselves or how we should be spending our time. Like a trapeze artist who must let go of one ring to catch the next, we must let go of the false in order to grasp the truth.

Reflection

How has your new way of seeing changed what has value in your world?

33.

The path to freedom leads from knowing the truth to living it. It covers the distance between our values and our actions. We undertake this journey within the maelstrom of everyday life, a field characterized by unwavering uncertainty, chaos, disappointments, and victories, all of which have the power to take our eyes off the prize. Mark Hall, a 20-year-old world-champion wrestler, sums it up this way: "All we can do is wrestle for seven minutes. We can't control what the refs do, we can't control what is going on around us; all we can control is our attitude and our effort." The third stage of enlightenment in Buddhism is where we learn respect for the simple virtues of everyday life. Kindness, enthusiasm, and equanimity are high on this list. Courage and humor aren't bad either. We come to prize those around us who model these virtues because we are learning that all we can control on the path to freedom is our attitude and our effort.

Reflection

Attitude and effort are the first skills we discover on the path. What are you learning about attitude and effort? Who around you is modeling the qualities you most wish to possess?

34.

Questioning the quest for gratification entails soul-searching reflection. However, questioning is not acting. The third stage is about walking the walk. We are allowing ourselves to be that which our hearts would have us be. The third stage flows from insight to action and from action back to insight. We choose a path of service that reflects our growing sense of connection to the human race. This service to others teaches us about ourselves. We reflect on these lessons, then bring them into our spiritual practice. As our spiritual practice deepens, we grow in our capacity to serve others. The path to freedom is a circle. It is a track. With each lap, we grow stronger.

I was drawn to the practice of yoga because it affirmed my sense of the sacred. How the divine shone from everything— each breath, each movement—a reminder of how we are held by life itself. This reflection led me to teach yoga. As I watch my students, I see my own struggles. I see them struggle to let go of fear. I see them struggle to let go of control. I see how burdened they are by the self they carry around. I see how important it is to put our burden down. I see how important it is to be on the path to freedom.

Reflection

Giving it away to keep it is part of the circle we are forming in our lives. How has helping others helped you?

35.

One morning after I watched *Homeland*, my meditation featured shadowy images of violence and urgency. When I have been in a conflict with someone, my meditation features numerous retellings of the event in which I am justified while the other person's positions are utterly demolished. Our body is made up of what we choose to feed it. Our mind is the same. Sitting in meditation, I can feel the effects of what I have consumed over the past 24 hours. Resting in stillness, it's all there for us to see. The tiredness from too little sleep, the way pizza has turned my stomach into a collapsed building, the way my resentments have boxed me into a small corner of my life.

The path to freedom is paved in truth. If we are careless, it will be like walking on hot coals. But it does not have to be this way. Mindfulness is a way to look closely at the truth without causing more harm, to see without blame. Twelve-step meetings are a way to look closely at the truth without causing more harm, to see without blame. A yoga pose is a way to look closely at the truth without causing more harm, to see without blame.

Reflection

Learning to see without blame is another skill we are developing. The next time you find yourself at a meeting, on a yoga mat, or on a meditation cushion, notice if you can see without blame. Blame will show up as tension in your body, which, if you look closely, will also be present in your mind. Can you keep looking but let go of that tension?

36.

B. K. S. Iyengar was the most influential yoga teacher of the 20th century. He was very good at what he did. One thing that made him so effective was his willingness to teach Westerners, and women in particular. His willingness to act beyond his culture's biases transformed the arc of his influence from local to global. The books he wrote on yoga have guided several generations of Yogis, offering millions of people a clarity on their paths to freedom they simply could not have had without his efforts. As a person of faith translating an Eastern spiritual tradition into an approach to life that made sense to me, I have found many of his teachings indispensable, none more so than his saying that "faith is a yoga vitamin."

In the attitude tool bag, faith has always loomed large for me. Faith is the antidote to the paralyzing reality of uncertainty. None of us ever know what is going to happen next. Yoga, meditation, and sobriety are all investments in a future we know nothing about. How do you invest with all of your heart in something that might not work out? Iyengar would say that we must learn the skill of faith.

Faith is a very difficult word, partly because it can seem, at best, intellectually flabby, and at worst, dishonest. To complicate an already difficult concept, faith has been used to justify countless forms of violence. This horrific reality is as disruptive today as it has been at any other point in human history. But there it is, the *F* word, *faith*. It is a skill we must possess if we are to invest one day at a time in an entirely new way of life. If nothing else, we must cultivate a faith in the possibility of sobriety for those who work toward it.

Reflection

What gives you faith? Who has modeled faith in your life in a way that inspires you?

37.

For the first 26 years of my life, I did not have faith in anything, but it wasn't really about having faith or not having faith. I had only the quest for gratification, pure and simple. I do not judge my young self for being this way; it was just the way things were. When I was sober, I began the process of questioning the chase. Before long I was faced with a dilemma. If I am not living to get something, what am I living for? What is worth getting out of bed in the morning for? I had to admit that in the quest for gratification, I was endlessly inventive in finding things I wanted to get. What did I want now? What did I value? What still had the power to move me?

The kindness that I was met with when I went to meetings moved me. The beauty of the natural world moved me. The desire to be a part of the beauty I was beginning to see in life moved me. When I looked a little more closely, I saw that I was talking about my heart. Life still touched my heart. My heart leaped at the beauty of it all—the forest, the nighttime sky, the world sobriety was revealing. The essence of this experience was gratitude. A person expresses gratitude for what already is. No getting, no chasing, just appreciation. I would stand in gratitude, meeting life with a faith in its beauty.

Reflection

As we get sober, we begin seeing the world as we once did before the numbing, depressing effect of our addiction. We look once again at the world with childlike wonder. Gratitude arises spontaneously. How does it feel to be moved by sober gratitude?

38.

The first principle of yoga is non-harming, and the second principle is honesty. We really could stop right there. Do no harm; live honestly. That would be enough. The rest of the skills that we will need for this journey will come to us if we have the capacity for honest, nonviolent self-reflection.

The first thing I needed to be honest about was my experience of addiction.

A. I was, in fact, powerless.

B. My powerlessness had made my life unmanageable.

C. I had no plan.

D. I should listen very closely to those who seemed to know what they were doing.

E. I should actually do what they suggested.

F. Failure to do so would leave me in the position of things getting worse.

G. I did not want to know what "worse" looked like.

The path may be paved with truth, but it is honesty that allows us to see it in the darkness. Honesty gives us the view.

Reflection

Attitude
Effort
Honesty
Clear seeing
Faith
Gratitude
Humor

These are the first skills we must possess on the path to freedom. Kindness and compassion will show up soon, but in early sobriety, we are like athletes training for an individual sport. We need to learn how to dedicate ourselves to a learning process. Seven skills for seven days: focus on one skill a day for a week, then do it again the next week, then the next, until learning these skills becomes part of your everyday life.

Three Views

For the last few essays of this chapter, I want to give each of our three traditions—yoga, 12-step, and the teachings of the Buddha—a chance to formally express their view.

Daily Reflections on Addiction, Yoga, and Getting Well

39.

Yoga has a name for the cause of our suffering, the Sanskrit word *avidya*. It means not seeing things as they are. *Vidya* means vivid, true knowledge, or seeing things in all their vibrant reality. Putting an *A* before the word *vidya* means that we are actively doing something to experience its opposite. *Avidya* means that we are actively participating in not seeing things as they are.

Avidya is the effect. The habits of the mind are the cause. These habits package reality in a series of shorthand intellectual artifacts in much the way that an automatic transmission turns five gears into "drive." This works fine as long as we have no reason to learn about the separate gears. If it turns out that the nature of the individual gears matters, then "drive" actively obscures the reality we must investigate.

Instead of "drive," we have had phrases like "getting high," "partying," or "drinking." These words masked a series of beliefs that justified a series of choices, which added up to addiction. Yoga takes the view that we must quiet the mind in order to notice the mind's habitual packaging of reality. Having noticed the distorting effect our mind is having, we learn to relax out of the effort it takes to package life. We learn to relax into connection with the present moment. This movement from a packaged view into a state of pure connection with the present moment is one of the fundamental transformations yoga makes possible. To connect to the present moment is to place your feet upon the path to freedom.

Reflection

My meditation teachers say that "the moment is self-liberating." They say that you can't bring the past, the future, or the self into the moment. What happens to your "story" when you connect with the present moment?

40.

The 12–step view does not focus on how we got into this mess as much as what the mess is and what we can do about it. The 12 steps start by saying that someone who needs treatment for addiction has become powerless over a behavior that is killing them. They go on to state that addiction has made the person's life unmanageable. A person beginning to attend 12-step meetings is confronted with potentially vexing questions. Am I actually powerless over my addiction? Is my life unmanageable? The newcomer is presented with a paradox. To get the power to heal, you must first admit that you do not possess it. You must surrender to win.

Having stated that the addict is powerless, the 12-step solution offers refuge in three specific behaviors.

1. Seeking God's aid (12-step is unapologetically theistic but not aligned with a specific religion)

2. Seeking the support of other addicts, meeting under the guidelines laid out in the 12 traditions that go along with the 12 steps

3. "Working the steps" by following the instructions laid out in the 12 steps

More than 80 years ago, Bill Wilson wrote that "rarely have we seen a person fail" who has actively found refuge in these three behaviors. This has also been my experience.

Reflection

Do the words powerless *and* unmanageable *sound accurate to your experience? Are you willing to try something new?*

41.

The Buddha taught that we suffer because we see backward. We think the impermanent is permanent; we think the unreliable is reliable; we think that which is not who we are is who we are. He went on to say that not only do we see backward, we vigorously defend our point of view. We cling to that which causes us to suffer. He taught that if we have learned to cling, we can learn to let go. He taught three behaviors that create the conditions in which letting go becomes increasingly available to us.

1. Cultivating wisdom (wise view)

2. Learning to be present without attachment

3. The practice of nonviolence in word, deed, and livelihood

Reflection

The Buddha taught that we are caught like a wheel in mud in a perspective that causes us to suffer. How can you tell when this is true for you? How does it feel to be caught like a wheel in mud? How do you get unstuck?

42.

My family and I went to the phenomenal play *Hamilton* yesterday. The poignancy with which this play depicts the hopes, dreams, and sorrows of humanity cannot be overstated. I cried during most of the scenes. I cried because it is a play about loss and what people do with it. In the final scene, Hamilton's wife describes the 50 years she spent alone after the death of her husband. How she interviewed the soldiers who served with him to better know the man she would never see again. How she honored him with acts of compassion, speaking out against slavery and creating a home for boys who had become orphans.

It is my view that recovery from addiction is about loss and what we do with it. We lose friends. We lose family members. We lose ourselves. We cannot get back what we have lost, but we can make our losses mean something. It is our only remaining option. We have life pulsing through us. Life never admits defeat. We have no choice but to find a way forward. The yoga, 12-step, and Buddhist traditions offer us a way.

Reflection

Write down what a "way forward" would look like for you. Who do you want to be? What kind of experience do you want to have?

43.

My heart has been broken by loss. My heart has been healed by love. I have watched my wife walk toward me in a white dress, a smile of joy on her face. I have seen my children take their first breath. I have held my son as he saw light for the first time. I have been in countless rooms where people have created a healing energy too beautiful to put into words. Life is worth the effort; the trick is not to quit.

If I were to offer one more skill for the "newcomer" it would be to be optimistic. When I was one year sober and things got hard, I would say to myself, "In five years, I want the problems of someone six years sober." I felt six years just had to be better than one. I wanted to be there for that. I wanted to be alive for the "It gets better" part.

Reflection

Connect to the part of yourself that hopes. What does it feel like to believe that it gets better? Why wouldn't it?

44.

There is a place between wanting and not wanting. I rest in it when I meditate. I cannot go there with my mind, or my heart, or my body alone. I must go there with all of them together. I must have the courage to let go of everything. This letting go of everything is the purest expression of yes. I sit quietly, saying yes to life with every fiber of my being.

Before I started using, life had already broken my heart. Using was just my way of admitting defeat. I had fallen down. Recovery has been about getting back up. Living sober is saying yes.

Reflection

How much of using was a way for you to cast your vote or to make a statement? What is the statement that you are making with your recovery?

Chapter Two

Intention

The purpose of this book is to show how three spiritual traditions have created a melody in my life. This melody has addressed the particular challenges I have faced as a recovering addict. For simplicity's sake, I am ascribing a particular emphasis to each tradition. Twelve-step meetings taught me to listen. Yoga poses taught me to feel. Meditation taught me to see. In this chapter, we will listen, feel, and see into the wholehearted, purpose-driven behavior captured by the term *wise intention*. What is the difference between being for, as opposed to against? What obstacles do we face when we attempt to give our all to something? What happens when we bring an unconflicted mind to bear on the matter at hand?

At one of my first meetings, I heard that Roy Rogers told his children to "believe in what you do and do it." This chapter concerns our ability to believe in what we do and do it.

45.

The Buddha sat in meditation in an effort to understand himself. He noticed that certain mind states led to suffering. He noticed that other mind states led to well-being. This understanding became known as wise view. Having understood what leads to suffering, having understood what leads to well-being, he made it his business to cultivate the mind states that lead to well-being. This decision became known as wise intention.

There is a moment in our recovery when we abandon the concept of being *against* anything in favor of being *for* something. This moment is when we come to understand the value of wise intention.

Reflection

Consider the word wholehearted. *Imagine the healing that must have taken place for an addict to be clean, sober, and wholeheartedly engaged in life. To live this way is the intention of recovery. Are you on board?*

46.

I spend a portion of each week coaching people individually. It is a way for me to teach what I need to learn. By listening to another person talk, I learn about my life. By feeling into someone's next level, I gain perspective on my next level. By teaching her how to take the next step, I learn how to take the next step. As I learn, I help others learn.

A woman once told me about how she wanted to support her young son and needed a job that would allow her to work from home. I saw the pain in her face as she talked about what she would do for her son. Nothing she could envision gave her any joy. She told me she'd had her chance at happiness and her time was past. Now it was her duty to help her son find the happiness that had eluded her. I asked her how she could help her son find something that she had not.

Reflection

All of us are teachers. Our life is our teaching. What is it you intend to teach? How will you teach it? Will you try to teach happiness while practicing despair? Will you teach joy while practicing love? What will you teach others about teaching?

47.

I have inherited my intention. Countless beings have taught me what courage looks like. Countless beings have taught me what love looks like. Countless beings have taught me grace in victory and defeat. Countless beings have taught me how to serve, how to provide, how to teach, how to love. I have inherited my intention. The beauty that stirs my heart was given to me. It has been a free gift. I cannot express the gratitude I feel, but I can try to live it one day at a time.

Reflection

Whose life has stirred your heart? What has this person taught you?

48.

I was not in a position to learn a great deal at my first 12-step meetings. I began to feel comfortable after a week or so. I knew which meetings had good coffee and where the bathrooms were. Eventually I began to be able to listen to what people were saying. Most people seemed to be saying extremely personal things about their drinking. It seemed that the admission that they were having a problem was part of it. This one did this, that one did that. It all made me uncomfortable, but I did not think anyone was making things up. These people had lived what they were talking about.

After they described their drinking, they would go on to say how heartfelt their desire to stay sober was becoming. This sincere desire manifested in a willingness to take action. I heard how "the program" works. I heard that because the program works, it was the speaker's intention to go to any lengths to follow it. By the time I had been sober for a month, I knew who was sincere in their desire to stay sober and who wasn't; I was able to recognize the resolve of wise intention when someone had it. Seeing this resolve in others helped me find my own.

Reflection

Who is modeling the resolve to stay sober for you in a way that is helping you find your own?

49.

The resolve I witnessed in meetings taught me that wise intention held equal measures of wisdom and compassion. The wisdom was expressed in the willingness to thoroughly examine the cause of suffering in one's life. The compassion was expressed in the willingness to stop harming oneself. The people in meetings had internalized oppression in a multitude of forms. This person had been oppressed because of her gender, this one because of her religion, this one because of her sexuality, this one because her parents knew no other way. Whatever form the oppression had taken, the bottom line was that people who come to 12-step meetings had learned to attach little or no value to their own well-being. The intention to stop harming themselves was radical. The intention to stop harming themselves was the beginning of the end of a process in which suffering was handed down from one generation to the next. The intention to stop harming themselves was changing the course of human history. Sitting in church basements on shabby metal chairs drinking bad coffee, I watched people changing the world by changing their intention.

Reflection

Two forms of willingness to change the world exist: the willingness to look closely at the cause of suffering in your life and the willingness to stop harming yourself. Don't try to do this alone. Find people who will laugh with you as you change the world. Who are these people in your life today?

50.

Looking closely at something reveals that you are looking at a verb, not a noun. An apple is a process, a river is a process, the sky is a process. Listening, feeling, seeing are processes. Looking closely is a process. Learning is a process.

When you first learn about a yoga pose, it appears to be a noun: "Today we will learn about triangle pose." You think, *Good enough, I will now do the noun* triangle. Then you look closely. The way the pressure of your front foot translates into the experience of the ankle is a process. There is no one thing. There is a series of sensations that never ends until you leave the pose. This series of sensations in the foot-ankle relationship affects the experience of the front hip, creating another series of sensations that does not end until you leave the posture. Once you leave the posture, you discover a "triangle echo" in the body. This echo will be present in the next pose for a while. The temporary nature of that echo is a part of the series of sensations that is the next pose. This is how my teacher described the relationship between karma and reincarnation. An echo of our past lives exists in our present one.

As you look closely at the experience of your body, you discover a process that is continually unfolding, a process that can be pleasant or unpleasant, depending on the skill with which you participate. This is wise understanding. Wise intention is the decision to participate in the process in a way that is enjoyable.

Reflection

Look closely at something. Using the sense that fits best—the taste of a bite of food, the sound of birds outside, the feeling of motion in the body while riding on a train or in a car—feel how life presents itself to us as a process that unfolds within the space of our awareness. Feel how we are the sky and life is the weather.

51.

The willingness to stop harming ourselves is one of the most important things we will ever cultivate. It is also a process that never ends. Looking closely at the choices we make from day to day, from moment to moment, we discover a process, a series of patterns. The cultivation of wisdom is the willingness to see a pattern through to discover which patterns lead to suffering, which patterns lead to well-being. People find it easier to do this together. In groups that are successful, you spend some time learning from others and some time observing your own experience. Together, you learn to observe. Together, you learn to be honest about what you are observing. However, this is not enough.

Being honest takes courage. Taking action takes more courage. In groups that are successful, you spend some time being inspired by others' courage and some time inspiring others with your courage. In the places where people are learning to be brave, you discover that courage is something you choose to honor your heart. The people who have found the courage to honor their heart stand out because they have embraced the intention to do no harm, one day at a time. These courageous ones have found it necessary to begin the process of non-harming with how they treat themselves.

Reflection

When you look closely, the decision to stop harming yourself is a leap of faith, a leap that requires courage. Who is helping you with this? What are you willing to do to get that help?

52.

Wise intention is informed by hard experience. We have held on to our addiction until we could not hold on anymore. The years of persisting on a path of suffering leave their mark. There is the physical evidence: the missing teeth, spouses, children, and bank accounts. But there is another legacy. We have had our hearts broken only to find them still there in the morning—broken, betrayed, yet still beating, still pointing us in the direction of love, tenderness, and gratitude. The intention of recovery begins on sacred ground, the place where there is no hope yet hope still exists. To know that possibility still exists where there is none, to know that love still exists where there is none, to know that kindness still exists where there is none, to know that the sacred remains when all else is gone—*this* is the legacy of those who survive addiction. *This* is the wisdom that informs the intention of recovery.

Reflection

What has it been like to lose hope, only to discover that hope hasn't lost you?

53.

The sacred remains when all else is gone. This is why everything has to go: so that we can see what we have been standing on all this time. In the gentle quiet that holds us at the end of the struggle, we look down to discover the path to freedom beneath our feet. Wisdom is seeing what is being offered. Compassion allows us to go on one more adventure.

Reflection

Do you see that you are standing on the path to freedom? Have you given yourself permission to go on the adventure of a lifetime?

54.

In order to teach yoga, I had to learn its purpose. To have a purpose, you must have an end in mind. The purpose of yoga is to deliver an experience of living that is free from suffering. The end is the end of suffering. I teach a set of disciplines whose purpose is freedom. With this understanding, I do not have to look far for my intention. My role is to guide people into a functional relationship with the disciplines of yoga so that they may use them to set themselves free.

When I guide students toward the felt experience of the breath, I suggest that they "slow the breath down enough to be able to feel it." I am not telling them how slow the breath should be. I am not telling them how to feel the breath. These are skills they are learning to set themselves free. If I do that work for them, I will not have served my purpose. Intention takes understanding and draws a thin line. On one side of the line, we find all that is not ours to do, live, or have. On the other side, we find a humble duty that must be taken up and lived with every fiber of our being.

Reflection

The Buddha said that every soul that awakens carries 10,000 souls with it across the river of suffering. Is getting sober enough for you? Can you be content with this duty?

55.

My meditation teachers say that your goal is the mountain that you are climbing. Your intention is the manner in which you take each step up the mountain. Having a goal points you in a direction and helps you to stay on course. Being clear about your goal lends an economy of effort to the way you use your time, organize your company, teach your classes, or raise your children. Clarity concerning one's purpose is essential to the success of any endeavor.

The role of intention is to translate one's purpose into a lived reality. If a goal organizes, an intention informs. An intention places the whole of our heart's desire into the space between the in breath and the out breath.

Reflection

If the mountain is sobriety, how do you wish to climb it? Name three qualities that you wish to bring to each step.

56.

My 20s were spent learning to live from the inside out. As an active addict, I had placed my faith in the way things looked. I had worked extremely hard to gain the appearance of success. The manner in which I put these symbols of success into place was irrelevant. It was all about the goal. By the time I got sober, I had little left to show for my attempts at looking good. In addition to having nothing left, seeming a way I did not feel no longer meant that much to me. Sobriety had slowed my life down enough for me to feel it. This fundamentally changed the way I defined success. I no longer wanted my life to look good. I wanted it to feel good.

This new understanding led to a new intention. I wanted my efforts to add up to self-respect. From this perspective, I was able to see that the form my life was taking from one moment to the next was temporary. The lasting benefit I could gain from whatever moment I was in would be what I learned from it. Moreover, I realized that I could decide what I wanted to learn within any given situation. I could practice courtesy, or follow-through, or kindness, or consistency (personal attributes I needed to work on in early recovery) whether I was attending a course, waiting tables at a restaurant, or greeting newcomers at a 12-step meeting. The role of intention in my life was to put me in charge of who I was learning to be, one day at a time.

Reflection

Who are you learning to be? What are you choosing to learn, one day at a time?

57.

Once I shift my gaze from a goal to an intention, I find myself looking at a verb, not a noun. A goal can be a trophy resting on a shelf; an intention is a process inviting us to show up a little better today than we were yesterday. To help me with this, my meditation teachers taught that a commitment to an intention is like a commitment to learning to ride a bicycle. When we commit to learning to ride a bicycle, we are not saying that we will never fall off the bicycle. We are saying that we commit to getting back on whenever we fall off. We are committing to a quality of heart that is steady, consistent, and content to get back on the bicycle until we have learned to ride it.

Reflection

The courage of recovery is not the courage of one who has never failed. The courage of recovery is the courage of one who is willing to fail over and over again until she succeeds. Who has that courage in your life? When have you demonstrated that courage?

58.

Yoga teaches us to find the quality of heart, the quality of being, that is content to work with the time that we have, the resources that we have, the health that we have, the body that we have, the circumstances that life has given us to achieve our goals. The Yogis take it for granted that everyone has to deal with too little time, too few resources. Everyone has to work without enough information; everyone has to accept heartbreaking setbacks. And these are just our external circumstances. Any time spent in honest self-reflection reveals a host of challenges that we would rather not have. So it is not a coincidence that whenever I go on a meditation retreat I discover other students have taped a particular saying in strategic spots throughout the facility. Sometimes I find this saying taped over a dishwasher or over the sink used for scrubbing pots and pans. Sometimes I discover it on a desk in the office or in a cubby where you put your shoes before entering the meditation hall. Whenever I spend time meditating with other Yogis, I will find this saying reminding us to be content to work with things as they are.

Do what you can, with what you have, where you are.

— THEODORE ROOSEVELT

Reflection

The underlying belief is that you will always find what you need on the path to freedom, so stop fretting and get busy.

59.

They say that faith is where you place your heart. As an active addict, I did not know where to place my heart so I would often lose it. I was a quitter, though I never would have described myself that way. I had won wrestling championships, I had earned academic honors, I had passed the Army's most difficult training. Yet I was a quitter because I did not know where to place my heart. My heart had no home. The people who taught me how to stop getting drunk created a sacred space with their presence, which I trusted entirely. It was within the circle they created that I found a place for my heart. It was within this circle that I learned how to give my heart entirely to something. Since then, I have been challenged, but I have never lost my heart.

Reflection

Have you found a place for your heart? If not, what would this place look like? Feel like? What would it mean to give your whole sober heart to something?

Wise Intention Defined

The type of intention that will serve us on the path to freedom is described in some detail by each of the three spiritual traditions that create the melody of my recovery.

Someone practicing this type of intention discovers:

A. That what you seek is close at hand

B. That what you seek is the freedom of being

C. That everything in your life is helping you to be free

Let's spend some time letting each tradition support you in this discovery.

60.

The Buddha sat in meditation in an effort to understand himself. For a while, he just observed. Eventually he recognized two basic patterns. One set of mental habits led to suffering; another led to freedom. With this information available, he defined a course of action for himself. He saw that fighting against negative patterns only strengthened them, so he made it his intention to embrace the mental habits that led to freedom.

These mental habits can be seen as skills for aligning with life, learning to go with the flow of a river as opposed to against it. The Buddha described the skills he used to go with the flow of life as being against the flow of ordinary human behavior. Ordinary human behavior results in suffering. The Buddha identified two skills of the heart and one skill of the mind that would allow him to live without suffering. These became his intention. They are:

1. Kindness

2. Compassion

3. Non-attachment

Reflection

Consider the implication of this short list. Two-thirds of it is treating yourself and others with care. Look closely at how little we need to know to be happy and how little is being asked of us.

61.

I first started hearing the word *non-attachment* in the 1990s. It felt culturally alien to me, something for other people, people who did not have my problems. My heart was heavy from a lifetime of loneliness; the last thing I thought I needed was non-attachment. Misunderstanding does not correct itself, so I lived in ignorance for quite a while. Nevertheless I was lucky. I was in the right place with the right people, doing the right things. This auspicious state of affairs allowed me to keep learning.

After my daughter was born, I began spending time with meditation teachers. They described non-attachment to me in a way that I could understand. They told me to sit and watch what happened when my mind grasped at something. To notice what attachment is like, then to soften back into the present, into the place between wanting and not wanting. What is it like to rest in non-attachment? They did not tell me what to think; they told me how to see for myself.

Reflection

How does it feel to crave? How does it feel to let go? Can you imagine letting go as a form of wisdom? Can you imagine letting go as a form of love?

62.

Attachment makes the case for non-attachment. We simply need to observe the chaotic and tragic role attachment plays in our lives to become firm in our intention to practice non-attachment. For at least 40 years I lived like someone who walked across their lawn only to step on a rake and end up in the ER—every day, year after year, believing that next time would be different. The rake was my belief that if only I got what I wanted, everything would be okay. This rake would get bigger when things started to go south. If it did not look like I was going to get what I wanted, I would want harder, more desperately. If what I wanted was threatened, it would loom ever larger as the thing that would make the difference, the thing that would provide the ultimate happiness.

I have spent most of my life never even suspecting that my attachment to getting what I wanted was causing the unhappiness in my life. Ask my family, ask my friends, ask my co-workers, ask anyone who has known me for more than 15 minutes, and they will tell you that when I am attached, I am a different person from who I am when I am not attached. I was the last person to know what everybody already knew about me. I sat in meditation for years suffering intensely over things not going my way, letting go only as a last resort when I could no longer bear sitting with my craving. I let go to be free from suffering. I had to. To hold on burned like fire. To let go was cool and soothing. I started to like letting go.

Reflection

What burns like fire? What is cool and soothing?

63.

In meditation we are learning to see something all the way through. To watch a sensation arise, change, fade, vanish. There is no need to make more out of something. There is no need to make less out of something. There is no reason to do anything but watch things come, change, and vanish over and over again. When it is time, we will understand the pattern. When it is time, we will know what something is like.

This is how we cultivate non-attachment. We simply observe attachment. Before long, we come to see the various states of attachment—the various waves of desire and aversion that sweep over us, the way these waves affect our perception. Craving makes us want something more than we want the truth, more than we want love, more than we want health, more than we want life. Sitting quietly, just watching, we come to know what attachment is like. Sitting quietly, just watching, we begin to lose our appetite for the mental state of attachment.

Reflection

Do you know what it is like to want something more than love, health, or life? Are you losing your appetite for that way of life?

64.

We begin the practice of non-attachment by falling out of love with attachment. We become less interested in winning the argument, getting the last word, or getting more than our fair share. We cross a line, and the quest for having is replaced by the quest for being. A good day starts being measured more by what we have given than what we have gotten. We start setting intentions around how we are showing up. Those of us who pray start praying for virtues instead of outcomes. When people talk about how they are getting better at generosity or compassion, we find ourselves on the edge of our seats. We find ourselves willing to go to any length to learn how to love well.

Going to any length for me these days means spending time on meditation retreats each year. A day on a meditation retreat is a roller coaster of breakthroughs, setbacks, soreness, and spaciousness. By the evening, I have usually come to the end of what I can do by my own efforts. It is time for someone else to carry the ball. Sitting quietly in California twilight, a Yogi starts teaching. She has spent her life learning what she is now sharing. She is not talking about getting what she wants. She is talking about being who she was born to be. As her words find my heart, I am no longer tired or defeated; I am on the edge of my seat.

Reflection

What gets you to the edge of your seat these days?

65.

For a while I could not understand the relationship between mindfulness and kindness or compassion. There was this cold mental discipline, and then there were these squishy heart practices that felt like nothing more than being nice. I tried to develop mindfulness, but I found that until I could hold something with the kind heart of compassion, I could not understand it, whether it was a behavior or a person. Without love, there is no possibility of understanding. Love allows us to see things as they are.

After several years of sobriety, I began working with young people who had had a hard time. It was my first opportunity to help others as I had been helped. It was my first chance to say thank you for all that had been given to me. The goal was to support a child into choosing life once again. The process was for a child to succeed often enough that she would start to believe in herself. As they approached the goal, you'd start to see a light in their eyes. Seeing that light emerge changed me forever.

We fall back into love with life one small, ordinary moment at a time. Watching these young people taught me how life happens, how miracles happen, how lives are saved, how lives must be lived. The love I felt for these children let me see how miracles happen.

Reflection

Attachment is another way of saying we are the center of things by which all things should be measured. Love offers us another way to measure. How has love changed how you see?

66.

To value non-attachment, we must first understand the suffering attachment causes. Once we have understood how attachment is affecting us, we will have to abandon judging ourselves for the habit of attachment. In the case of addiction, we must be willing to let ourselves off the hook for a pattern that nearly killed us. In the space of our own kindness, we will learn the difference between a person and a behavior.

First we learn to see the problem without judgment. Then we learn to see ourselves without judgment. Something new becomes available to us. We wake up from a dream in which there was no hope or possibility to see that there is a way. Amidst the ruins of our active life, there is a path leading to an entirely new existence. Looking closely at the path, feeling its invitation, we put our burden down and start walking.

Reflection

What is it like to see a new possibility? What is it like to smile at the joy of it? What is it like to let your burden down? What has it been like to start walking in the right direction?

67.

To unlearn the habit of attachment is the hardest thing we can do. Recovering from addiction is this very same challenge in an extreme form. Like someone caught in a riptide, the addict cannot swim to safety by simply swimming harder. The power necessary to get to shore comes from three sources.

A. **Wisdom:** We must have the wisdom to let the current take us to safety.

B. **Willingness:** We will need the current of addiction or attachment itself. The very process that is trapping us has the power to bring us to safety if we are willing to let it.

C. **Heart:** When we are caught in a riptide, we cannot swim toward the shore, however close it appears. Caught in a riptide, we must let it take us away from shore toward a safety we cannot see or understand. This will take heart.

Reflection

Getting to safety is one-third wisdom, one-third willingness, and one-third heart. When I feel into these qualities, I sense a life worth living, an honest life, a sincere life. Are you up for this?

68.

When I teach a student to move mindfully, I get specific. I tell her to move smoothly. Moving smoothly requires a form of attention that delivers the experience of mindfulness. Over time, she will find herself bringing this quality of attention into everything she does because mindfulness is a form of paying attention that is suited to every occasion. Once she is moving smoothly, I tell her to add kindness to the movement. Having felt smooth, she is ready to feel the difference kindness makes. Everybody can feel kindness in their movements. Everybody gets excited when they do.

As a teacher, I love this kind of dramatic experience because students tend to remember it. Years later, students who have had this type of experience will return to it when they get on their yoga mats. When they do, they discover that smoothness is connected and kindness is intelligent. This is a form of paying attention that is suited to every occasion.

Reflection

Breathe smoothly. What is it like? Move smoothly. What is it like? Now as you move smoothly with the breath, add the intention to be kind to your body. What is the difference kindness makes?

69.

We practice a form of paying attention that is smooth and kind for a reason. We will need to connect with intelligence if we are going to be able to feel the difference between attached and non-attached participation. Noticing this difference provides us with the opportunity to choose. Not from regret or shame, but from self-care. Once we begin to practice non-attachment, the only mistake we can make is to stop practicing.

Reflection

When you feel yourself getting caught up in a negative mind state, slow down. Slow and deepen the breath. Slow and smooth out your movements. When things calm down a little, include the intention to be kind to yourself and others.

70.

I got sober young. My friends from that time were mostly other young people getting sober in their 20s. There was a special sort of relief that we felt when we were together. All of us had been traumatized as children. All of us had made things worse by trying to self-medicate. All of us carried the burden of shame for having been traumatized, for having been addicted, for having had to surrender, for having had to ask for help. None of us had expected to survive our addictions. There was a relief that we felt at having survived long enough to find a life worth living.

There was a hope. It was the hope that we could live usefully. It was the hope that we could walk humbly through a sober life. It was the hope that when our days were done we would die sober. There was a knowledge that living and dying sober mattered.

Reflection

The relief of recovery is good. Experiencing it with others is even better.

71.

There is a moment in our recovery when we admit that we cannot do anything about our situation by ourselves. This understanding can be a doorway to despair or it can lead to the help that we need. If it leads to getting help, we develop an intimate knowledge of what actually has the power to help a human being live her life. Having had this experience, we become both humble and useful.

Reflection

The shame we feel at having to ask for help makes it difficult for us to see the value of what we are learning about addiction and the impact our recovery will have on everyone we meet. Having admitted we can't do one thing, we doubt our ability to do anything. Do you understand how important your learning process is?

72.

Recovery is a restoration. As we are relieved of our addiction, we come to live usefully and walk humbly. The 12-step phrase is "a return to normal living." The galvanizing vision I received in my first months of sobriety was composed of hopelessly addicted individuals regaining their health, their faith, their natural capacities, and then returning to everyday life, all the better for having survived their addiction. I saw a global community operating invisibly on behalf of humanity's true potential. Actors, politicians, educators, parents, students moving through the world with a uniquely compassionate point of view, having had their lives given back to them by complete strangers. I wanted to be a part of this invisible army whose motivation was nothing less than pure gratitude. This is the intention that has guided my steps in recovery.

Reflection

When I think of the intention of recovery, I think of the words freedom, gratitude, *and* service. *What would be your words?*

73.

Bill Wilson began working with others in an effort to understand himself. He determined that without aid, he was powerless over his drinking. He came to believe that the aid of prayer combined with the support of other people like himself had the power to end his drinking. These insights became known as the first and second steps. Having understood the nature of his addiction, Bill Wilson made the decision to organize his life around the behaviors that had the power to set him free. This decision became known as the third step.

Wise view is an accurate analysis of the cause of suffering in our lives. Wise intention is the decision to follow up that analysis with action. For an addict seeking help, the first three steps of a 12-step program consist of wise view and wise intention. At a meeting, these teachings are broken down by people who have used them effectively. From many voices, you will hear the nature of your condition and what you can do about it.

Reflection

An important 12-step phrase is "Let go absolutely." Wise intention in a 12- step program encompasses the willingness to let go absolutely. It is considered wise to let go of the old way of living in order to learn a new one.

74.

The Buddha was deeply moved by the suffering he saw in the world around him. This suffering drove him to find an answer. I was deeply moved by my own suffering, but I could not do a thing about it. My story does not include a quest for knowledge or a quest for freedom. At the end of my drinking, I was roadkill on the highway to the hell that is addiction. Mine is not the Buddha's story. I needed more help than he did. I needed people who understood me better than I did. I needed a well-worn path. The only trail I was capable of blazing was to my next meeting. Because of the efforts of countless other addicts, the willingness to show up was enough.

A 12-step meeting supports people in the exact same journey the Buddha embarked on. The difference is the condition they are in when they begin their journey. Accounting for this difference is how the 12-step community radically changed human potential.

Reflection

An important 12-step phrase is "Keep coming back." All that is required of us is the willingness to show up. The path is well worn. Just keep coming.

75.

When it became time for me to develop a meditation practice, I chased it the way I chased sobriety. I attended meditation retreats the way I had attended meetings. It was a good choice, one of the best I have ever made. During this time, I went to fewer meetings. I had young children and a business to run, time was in short supply. As my children got older, the middle of my days started to open up. I found my way back to more regular meetings. In meditation I had learned to sit quietly and watch my mind. The idea is if you sit quietly, watching, the habits of the mind will reveal themselves to you. Ultimately you are meant to watch the mind and then apply the skills you are taught by your teachers in real time.

Sitting quietly at a meeting after some time away, I watched a circle of people having a remarkably effective discussion about the habits of their minds. These people would name a habit of the mind, then describe how they were learning to meet this habit with the skills they were gaining in meetings. It wasn't that I had come full circle. It was that I saw the table at which we were sitting—some people on this side, others on that side, all having the same meal.

Reflection

A popular 12-step saying is that recovery is an inside job. Watch the mind and apply the skills. What does it mean to you that the solution is entirely internal?

76.

In the final days of my active addiction, my disease felt like a fire that was burning out of control. My first few days of sobriety were spent reflecting on the ashes of my former life. I was young, well educated, and my life was over. It felt as if I had completely failed at life. The flames of my addiction had burned a circle around me in which nothing could live, across which nothing could pass. This circle became the place where I would do the inner work of early recovery. Bereft of any meaningful "outer work," I was able to devote my time to what was still left—my health, my heart, my mind, my soul.

For a precious few years, it was not possible for me to "succeed" in any traditional sense of the word. I could not have dissipated my energy in the pursuit of importance if I had wanted to. In the midst of a society consumed by the quest for gratification, I began a personal search for meaning. Living in shabby apartments, holding down low-paying jobs, I discovered a profound form of wealth. It came to me not in the form of possessions but in sensations—the sensation of inner peace, the sensation of gratitude, the sensation of self-respect, the sensation of empathy, the sensation of compassion. These were the forms of wealth I discovered when all else was gone. The destruction my addiction had wrought in my life had freed me from anything that would compete with what was now my life's work: walking the path to freedom.

Reflection

When I took my first job as a healer, my personal income was cut in half. My 12-step sponsor said, "You must not have needed the money." He was right. How has the destruction of your active addiction created the space for you to do the work of recovery?

Barn's burnt down . . . now I can see the moon.

— MIZUTA MASAHIDE

77.

Sobriety is the light of the moon by which we discover ourselves, each other, and our purpose. Gathering in moonlit circles, we sing the song of our hearts.

Reflection

The next time you are in a gathering of recovering people, feel the song in your heart. What is your heart's intention?

78.

Seeking to understand yoga, the ancient scholar Patanjali wrote down the Yoga Sutras, which had been passed down orally for countless generations. He believed that when the mind moves, it turns away from the present, whereas when the mind is still, it connects to the present. He felt that turning away from the present distorts our perception, whereas connection to the present allows us to gain vivid, true knowledge. With these tenets in mind, he concluded that the purpose of yoga is to bring the mind to stillness. The purpose of yoga is connection.

Recovery is the movement from craving to connection.

Reflection

To experience what is meant by connection, just sit still. Become upright and relaxed at the same time. Find the middle between the effort of being upright and the ease of relaxing. Notice that as the body finds the middle, the mind finds the moment.

79.

Stopping the mind may seem like an impractical exercise for addressing the problem of addiction until we reflect on what the mind is like when we are caught up in craving. Consider for a moment the mind states of active addiction. Even the briefest reflection on "what it was like" reveals a clear and present need to develop a better relationship with our own minds.

Fortunately, yoga does not instruct us to "stop the mind." It teaches us how to pay attention in a way that allows the mind to flow in a state of connection from one moment to the next. It begins with a simple instruction: move from thinking to feeling. As you are sitting, know that you are sitting. As you are breathing, know that you are breathing. Instead of stopping anything, we are being invited to start connecting.

Reflection

As you sit, know that you are sitting. Bring gentle awareness into the body. As you breathe, know that you are breathing. Bring gentle awareness to the breath. Practice connection.

80.

Recovery is the movement from craving to connection. In yoga, we practice this movement over and over again, day after day, until it becomes second nature. Whatever I am doing—whether in conversation, on my mat or cushion, teaching or learning, at dinner with my children or spending time with friends, breathing in and breathing out—a part of me is aware of the level of tension in my body. If my body is resting in a certain way, I know I am in a state of connection. When my body contracts, however slightly, I know I have begun to lean into craving. When I notice the tension of craving in my body, I relax back into connection. If that is not available to me, I take a breath in. As I breathe out, I relax back into connection. Yoga has taught me how to bring recovery into each step I take.

Reflection

Practice taking a long, slow, easy breath in. As you let it out, relax into the felt experience of your body. Do this for as long as you want. Do this often. Do this until you know that ease and connection are a part of you, like your sense of humor or generosity.

81.

Yoga is an expression of our desire to regain our connection to this timeless moment. The act of connecting to the present moment has become an art of yoga because we have developed the habit of disconnection. The act of connecting to the present moment has become a practice of yoga because the state of disconnection leads to suffering. We connect to the present moment through the senses in the way that someone testing the bathwater for her child becomes entirely present for the feel of the water. In order to listen, feel, taste, smell, or see, we become still and alert. We focus our attention until we have made a connection with something that exists in this timeless moment. Yoga reinforces our ability to connect to something that exists in this timeless moment.

As a person in recovery, going to yoga was the kind of thing people like me did, so I did it. My introduction to yoga was through a series of movements and physical postures. I would go to yoga class to do these movements and postures to get the benefits of them, as I vaguely understood them. Go-do-get. With practice, yoga became a way I felt in my body, a way to be in the moment. It became a way to give my undivided attention to living sober. Feel-be-give.

Reflection

What does it mean for an addict in recovery to move from the habit of "go-do-get" to "feel-be-give"?

82.

To listen, feel, taste, smell, or see, we choose a certain kind of mental stillness that allows us to focus on something specific. Once we have made the connection, we examine it to understand it. How does the wind sound moving through the trees at night? How does it smell? How does it feel on my skin? How does it feel to be here on this night, standing on this forest floor, connecting to air moving in this way? Connecting in this way, we come to know what is true about the wind, or how a soup tastes, or how a friend's smile changes us after a hard day.

Yoga breaks down the process of connection into two specific skills. These skills combine to give us a way to be in connection. These skills combine to create an intention. As we connect to the world around us and within us, it is our intention to "neither abandon nor coerce our experience." This intention manifests as intimacy with life itself. In yoga, we learn that intimacy happens when we have let go of control, when we have committed to neither coercing nor abandoning our experience, our hearts, our minds, our loved ones, our community, or our planet.

Reflection

The phrase my meditation teachers taught me is "I will neither abandon nor coerce my experience." Bring this into your body. Feel your breath moving through your body without coercing it or abandoning it.

83.

The first of the two skills of Yogic connection is called *abhyasa*. It is the will to align and repeatedly realign to the present moment. It is the opposite of turning away from the present moment. As we practice *abhyasa*, we are learning to turn toward the moment. I explain this skill in two parts:

1. Choosing to connect to the present moment

2. Resting in that connection

We turn toward life. We choose connection, but we are not coercing that connection. Instead, we are learning to rest in it.

Reflection

Choose connection by sitting with a long spine and an open heart. Then rest in that connection by maintaining the effort it takes to be upright and openhearted while letting go of any extra effort in your body. Connect to the present by sitting upright and openhearted without an ounce of extra effort. Feel the depth of the letting-go process.

84.

We choose connection by shifting our attention from thinking to feeling, smelling, tasting, hearing, or seeing. For those of us who are willing to make a wholehearted effort, the contrast could not be more profound. In one moment, we are in our heads experiencing life through the filter of our story. In the next moment, we are back on earth taking in the profound richness of being alive. This unfiltered experience of being alive cannot be captured in words; it must be experienced directly. This is why Patanjali, the author of the Yoga Sutras, said that yoga is the mind in stillness. He did not try to explain what is perceptible when the mind is in stillness because it is literally indescribable.

We choose connection in the way we make any other choice. We choose connection to get peace or to escape suffering. However, as we move into connection, our thoughts of getting or avoiding are left behind. Stepping into the sunlight, we forget the rain.

Reflection

Connection *is another word for* intimacy. *In yoga, we are practicing an intimate connection with life. It is said that we cannot bring our attachments into the moment. Try it. See if you can connect intimately with the sound of birds or the taste of an apple while planning, worrying, regretting, comparing, or doing anything other than intimately connecting with what is true here now.*

85.

Abhyasa is choosing connection, the second skill, *vairagya* is resting in connection. Patanjali defined *vairagya* as the ability to "allow phenomena to arise and pass without reacting." Because of his choice of words or an error in translation, *vairagya* is often described as non-reaction. This definition tends to confuse new students into the belief that *vairagya* is a sort of white-knuckled equanimity in which you learn to never react to anything. The actual skill of *vairagya* is the ability to observe without external or internal commentary. This is an intimate form of observation in which we rest in connection much like a child rests her hand in yours as you walk together. We allow the experience in. The sound, the taste, the sensation is received, savored, seen, known directly. I learned from the Zen tradition that this form of knowing is only possible once we have abandoned the desire to gain from it. We are simply knowing because it is our nature to connect, savor, and know.

A part of knowing is the moment something arises. Sound arising is like this. A part of knowing is the moment something is here. Sound is like this. A part of knowing is the moment when something vanishes. Sound fading is like this. A part of knowing is the moment when something has passed. Silence is like this. As we practice the skill of *vairagya*, we rest easy in the process of knowing what life is like.

Reflection

Sit quietly and listen. Find a sound, from the birds outside or passing cars or a nearby conversation. Listen to the sounds arise, change, then vanish. Listen to the silence. Listen to the next sound. Watch phenomena arise and pass. See if you can listen without commentary.

86.

Vairagya is a form of paying attention in which we neither coerce nor abandon our experience. In a yoga pose, we learn to take an action without an ounce of extra effort. In *vairagya* we learn to pay attention without an ounce of extra effort. Attachment of any kind is extra. In *vairagya* we are learning to pay attention without attachment. This was a process for me in which I learned to let go of a series of mental habits. Each was important in its own right, but ultimately, until I learned to let go of all of them, I was still holding on to something. As I attempted to observe without commentary, I had to unlearn the habits of:

1. Seeing whatever was happening as a commentary on "me"

2. Defending the idea of "me"

3. Fixing the idea of "me"

4. Judging whatever was happening in terms of how it related to "me"

Reflection

Listen to the silence and feel your mind becoming silent. Feel your mind become empty of the self.

87.

Once we have learned to place our attention on the present, we learn to rest in connection. When I lead a yoga class, the expectation is that we will be able to rest in connection for several breaths; then the habit of the mind to wander will kick in. This is when I give my next cue. My cueing sounds like this, punctuated by pauses of three breaths each. The goal is to find the music between the notes:

> Become upright with a long spine . . . Notice that as your spine lengthens, your heart opens . . . Now begin the process of letting go . . . Balance the intention to be open-hearted with the intention to let go . . .

This goes on for the length of the class. These days, I teach only in workshop settings, so my yoga classes tend to approach two hours in length. The average yoga student finds no difficulty practicing like this for two hours straight.

Meditation is harder. We are on our own, with no one telling us what to do every four or five breaths. We have to think on our feet. We have to work it out. We have to learn how to be our own teacher. In wrestling, when someone gets better quickly, they say the athlete has made "jumps." Meditation is where we make jumps because we are practicing the right disciplines and learning how to apply the disciplines in a way that is tailored to our specific needs. We are learning what choosing connection is like. We are learning what resting in connection is like. We are learning in this body, this breath, this mind, this heart.

Reflection

Take a seated position that balances effort and ease. Find the middle. Then rest in the middle. Notice that as your body finds the middle, your mind finds the moment.

88.

The Buddha, Bill Wilson, and Patanjali practiced in an effort to free themselves. They discovered what imprisoned them and what had the power to set them free. Having understood this, it became their intention to embrace the behaviors that led to freedom. They found that they could not fight the wind nor push the river. They had to abandon the fight. They had to let go absolutely. Each step they took on the path to freedom would have to be taken with undivided attention. Each step would have to be taken with kindness. If they lived with one mind, one heart, their feet would find the way to freedom.

Reflection

My experience of sobriety is easy and joyful. I came to this ease, this joy, by way of an unconflicted mind and an unconflicted heart. This clarity of heart and mind comes from the clarity of my purpose, which arises from the steadfastness of my intention *to embrace the disciplines of freedom.*

89.

Early recovery is an intensely private struggle. Fighting against long odds from a position of weakness, we rally what heart, wits, and courage we have left to face a challenge whose outcome will be either life or death. We will endure most of this struggle entirely alone. Twelve-step meetings give us an hour or two a day when we can sit around the campfire, tell our stories, laugh, and learn before we go back out again to choose the life we want. On my 365th day of sobriety, I went to a noon meeting that was attended by 60 to 70 addicts, most of whom had watched me walk through my first year. I told my story that day to honor myself, my community and to say thank you to the God of my sobriety. I was raw—my future was uncertain, my past weighed heavy on my heart—but I had done something that mattered and there were people who cared. When I told my story on that day, it was to a community that felt like family in a place that felt like home.

Reflection

It's okay to need someone to care. It's okay to need someone to bear witness. It's okay to set aside time to be seen. Meetings are ways to do that for yourself; you simply need to be willing to be vulnerable.

90.

The addicted person is a traumatized person, which is to say some-one who is no longer at home in her own body. The body has be-come a vessel for pain and relief, that is all. It can bring pain, or it can bring relief. Either way, it is no more of a friend than anything else in a life that has not worked out. Coming back to the body is an intensely private struggle. Fighting against long odds from a position of weakness, we rally what heart we have left, what wits we have left, what courage we have left to face a challenge we know next to nothing about. We will endure most of this struggle entirely alone. Yoga classes give us an hour or two a day when we can trust our bodies again, learn from them, care for them, before we go back out again to choose the life we want.

Toward the end of my first year as a yoga teacher, I was leading a class in a friend's living room. The students were soccer players who needed something to do together during the cold months of winter. I taught them how to be still, to move, to breathe in a way that felt safe and sacred. I taught them that the body is a sanctu-ary we enter to spend time in the presence of the truth.

Reflection

The body is a sanctuary we enter to spend time in the presence of the truth. Go to class. Keep going. You've got this!

91.

At meetings, the mind is often described as a scary neighborhood that should not be entered alone. This gets a lot of laughs for all the right reasons, but we can't live as if the mind is unsafe. We must befriend the mind, which is to say we must learn to meditate. Reclaiming our inner life is an intensely private struggle. Fighting against long odds from a position of weakness, we rally what heart we have left, what wits we have left, what courage we have left to face a challenge few among us have even considered. We will endure most of this struggle entirely alone. Meditation retreats give us some time each year to sit quietly with our own heart, our own mind, connecting to nature, connecting to truth before we go back out again to choose the life we want for ourselves.

When I go to a meditation retreat, I arrive several hours before it begins to sign in, get my room and service position. Once I am settled, I usually go for a hike through the hills that surround the center. Coming down from the hills before dinner, I enter the meditation hall. It is usually empty. For more than 20 years, people have meditated in this hall. We have sat for hours, days, weeks, months, slowly bringing attention back into the fullness of our lives. As we expand our awareness, we discover the silence and stillness of eternity holding us. When we place our attention on silence, its presence intensifies. When we place our attention on stillness, its presence intensifies. Twenty years of practice have created a vortex of sacred stillness, a vortex of sacred silence in this hall built by my teachers. Walking into the meditation hall, I pause to feel the power of what we have created by listening to our heart's intention. Then I take a seat in an empty hall to be filled with peace.

Reflection

The mind is spacious peace, a vessel for wisdom. Go on a retreat. Keep going. You've got this!

Chapter Three

Truth

The role of the truth in recovery from addiction cannot be overstated. Unfortunately, we have not cultivated much of a relationship to it on our way to our next fix. In recovery, we need to develop a sense of what the truth looks, feels, and sounds like. We need to become adept at seeing, feeling, and listening for what is true here, now, then live from that truth. This chapter is dedicated to how that learning process was made possible for me by yoga, meditation, and the 12-step process.

92.

The Buddha sat in meditation in an effort to understand himself. He noticed that certain behaviors led to a harmonious existence. He noticed that other behaviors led to suffering. Having understood this, it became his intention to abstain from the behaviors that led to suffering. Having understood this, it became his intention to practice the behaviors that led to a harmonious existence. This decision became known as *sila*.

There is a moment in our recovery when we realize that true ambition is the desire to live usefully and walk humbly in harmony with all beings. It is at this point that we come to understand the true meaning of the ancient concept of *sila*.

Reflection

Make a short list of behaviors that bring you into internal and external harmony. Make a short list of behaviors that bring you out of harmony.

93.

When it came time for the Buddha to teach the concept of *sila* to his students, he broke it down into three basic forms of behavior: wise speech, wise action, and wise livelihood. Each was a spiritual practice in its own right. Each was an inquiry into the establishment of harmony. Wise speech focused specifically on our relationship to the truth. Can we live in harmony with the truth? Wise action focused specifically on the role our conduct plays in our inner life. Which actions create mental and emotional harmony? Which actions lead to mental and emotional suffering? Wise livelihood concerns the role we play in our communities. How can we support ourselves in a way that is in harmony with those around us? How can we support ourselves in a way that does not cause suffering for ourselves or others?

The idea was that a portion of our spiritual life would take place on sacred ground, and the remainder would take place in the hustle and bustle of everyday life. We could learn part of what we needed to know about life by stepping out of it to focus on practice, and the rest by stepping into life in order to learn by living. *Sila* turns our everyday life into a sacred learning space.

Reflection

Reflect on each of these areas of your life: speech, action, and livelihood. Reflect on the intention that motivates your behavior. Now consider the intention of harmony.

94.

When teaching the concept of *sila*, the Buddha offered his students two types of practice: *varitta*, the practice of abstaining from unwholesome behaviors, and *caritta*, the practice of embracing wholesome behaviors. Harming is avoided; kindness is practiced. Stealing is avoided; generosity is practiced. Ill will is avoided; compassion is practiced. Harmful sexual activity is avoided; the wise use of our sexual energy is practiced. The use of intoxicants is avoided; sobriety is practiced.

I have lived this way for 27 years. Though my track record has been average, the attempt has been magnificent. Any step in a direction toward health has been its own reward. Each day that I let go of something that does not serve me has touched my heart with gratitude. Each day that I practice a skillful habit has touched my heart with gratitude. Making the effort puts me in harmony with life itself. Making the effort is enough.

Reflection

What does it feel like when you make the effort?

95.

Having *understood* the behaviors that lead to suffering, it is our *intention* to practice the behaviors that lead to harmony. These behaviors are the disciplines of *sila*. The first is wise speech.

The fact that we have understood why wise speech matters implies that we have reflected on the suffering unwise speech has caused us over the years. For most of us, this is not a pleasant reflection. Rather, it is a cringe fest that represents the price addicts tend to pay for wisdom. In fact, this sort of reflection can lead to more suffering as we wish we hadn't done this or said that, but ultimately, as we reflect on the train wreck that is intemperate speech, we are forced into compassion. Never has there been anyone who can more readily say, "I didn't know that I didn't know" than an addict reflecting on her active behavior. So we embark on the journey of wise speech equipped with a heart made tender by the pain we have caused and the pain we have felt from words spoken in ignorance. We become truly grateful to have a chance to choose words spoken with kindness, words spoken with compassion and wisdom.

Reflection

Imagine friendships and families in which words do not cause harm.

96.

Neither my mother nor my father could ever bring themselves to say that I was good enough in behavior, attitude, or action. They were just being "honest" with me. They meant no harm; they simply could not bring themselves to say something that did not feel true to them. Their inability to appreciate themselves trapped them in a dynamic in which nothing their children did was ever enough.

My parents' predicament was that they wanted the best for their children but could not bring themselves to offer it. Our speech is but a reflection of our understanding. If our speech is to become wise, kind, and truthful, then we must be wise, kind, and truthful.

Reflection

Consider your parents' world, past and present, how that affected what they could or could not say to you. How are you like them now?

97.

The first time I can remember making a commitment concerning my speech was as a young military officer. At 24, I took over a 30-person infantry platoon guarding the border between East and West Germany in the midst of the cold war. I was very young, but my mission was very real. The men I worked for carried nearly unbearable burdens. The tasks they would perform in the event of war would cause the deaths of thousands of people regardless of who "won" the war. Within this extraordinary context, I questioned my addict's loyalty to lying.

Up until that point, I had practiced lying with an almost monastic devotion. I had grown up in a household where punishment was meted out with a hockey stick by an enraged adult. As an active child who transgressed often, there was no upside to honesty. I lied constantly. My lying took a toll on my inner life, but the alternative was significantly worse. Once I left my home, the stakes were lower, but I still gave no particular thought to whether or not what I said was true. I said what needed to be said to get what I wanted. Besides, I had developed a drinking habit that no one needed to know about.

While serving my country, assisting estimable elders as they carried a heavy burden, I considered the price of lying. It was not a lengthy process. Once I got to Germany, it was almost immediately clear that the people I worked for needed the truth from me as soon as I was in possession of it, no matter what it might cost me. The pain of looking bad to my superiors paled, in my estimation, to the pain of adding to my superiors' difficulties or letting my country down. For the first time in my life, as I decided whether to tell the truth or not, I included the effect my behavior would have on others. This is how the truth became far more attractive to me. I discovered a new form of courage. I no longer cared if things didn't work out for me, as long as I had done what was right.

Reflection

What was your relationship to the truth when you were growing up? What is it now? What has changed?

98.

During my years in the military, I learned that being someone whose word could be trusted was indispensable. My colleagues did not have to like me, but they had to be able to trust my word. Their lives depended on it. I saw how vulnerable everybody was, how they needed the truth in order to make the difficult choices their duty required. I saw how vulnerable I was to failing my heart. I went into the military to serve my country. I had taken an oath; I had given my word. Keeping my word was a verb, not a noun. Keeping my word was a process that unfolded in each conversation, each report. I learned that honesty was a form of courage. I learned that honesty was a form of faith.

Years later, my yoga teachers would remind us that our bodies are made of what we eat. What I learned during my years in the military but could not put into words at the time was that we are also made up of what we love. If we can keep our word to those we love, we grow stronger. If we break our word, we grow weaker. The military taught me the strength that comes from being true to your word. It was not long after this lesson that I became honest about my addiction.

Reflection

What helps you keep your word to your heart?

99.

Being someone whose word could be trusted became meaningful to me in the years before I got sober. It mattered to me that I had the courage to tell my commander the truth regardless of how it made me look. It mattered to have acted honorably. Without knowing it, I had begun to include my heart in my decision making. Even before I got sober, I had begun to recognize that true ambition was to live usefully and walk humbly. For this I will be forever grateful to the military.

Toward the end of my years in Germany, well into the process of discovering that *honor* is a verb, I showed up to work to discover that a soldier in the unit I led had died. At 19, he had been hit by a train while out for a night of drinking. I would spend the next week collecting his remains and accompanying his body home to his family. I acted as honorably as I could, which is to say that I put my heart into my duties. Showing up with heart as the family processed the alcohol-related death of their child was the end for me. It would be 10 more months before I got sober, but there would be no more months of the delusion that my drinking was working. Getting honest in the performance of my military duties had made it impossible for me to escape the truth that it was just a matter of time before my family would be processing my own alcohol-related death.

Reflection

I owe my life to this young addict because his death woke me up. Have there been addicts in your life whose death helped you wake up?

100.

After the funeral for the soldier who had died from his addiction, I began to get honest about my own addiction. I put a call in to a close friend to tell him about my drinking. During that call, I committed to telling my commanding officer about my drinking the next day, which I did. A few days later, I was honest about my drinking to the substance abuse counselors on base. The downside of this form of honesty was immediately apparent in that I continued to drink but now felt worse about it.

I had gotten honest, but the clouds hadn't parted. I still had my problems, but I no longer had guilt-free access to getting numb. Maybe getting honest was overrated? It turns out getting sober is a verb because getting honest is a verb. I had told my commanding officer that I had a problem, I had told my counselors I had a problem, but I had not determined for myself the exact nature of the problem. So I kept drinking to deal with the emotions that were coming up around my drinking.

I knew I had a problem, but I did not care enough to invest in the solution. I had admitted that I had a problem but had not accepted what that meant. The distance between admitting and accepting is a series of consequences that will end in death or truth. Those who survive accept a simple truth. Addiction only gets worse. If I cannot live with worse, my only alternative is to find a way to live sober.

Reflection

What did it take for you to move from admitting you had a problem to accepting what that meant?

101.

When we speak honestly about our private life, we are deliberately making ourselves vulnerable. This tends to feel pretty raw when we are new to it. Letting people know you have been drinking like a crazy person for years is a radical version of this dynamic. The sheer discomfort of this form of vulnerability has been enough to dissuade countless individuals from getting the help they need. Countless individuals have chosen death over vulnerability. This doesn't mean honesty is optional. A single-cell organism can protect itself or it can receive nutrients, but it can't do both at the same time. We can protect ourselves or we can grow.

My first few months of this kind of honesty were brutal. I felt utterly humiliated. The only time I felt the least bit okay was when I was alone or with other addicts in recovery. Initially I had the strength of the desperate. I was honest the way someone being chased by a horde of zombies would be honest about the need for help. As the months passed, I began to have a sense of what sobriety felt like. I was eating healthy food. I was getting a good night's sleep. I was exercising. I was experiencing waves of gratitude. I was looking forward to certain meetings. I could feel the path to freedom beneath my feet. Each time I was honest, I felt myself getting closer to the life I wanted to lead.

Reflection

What has been your experience of the relationship between honesty and freedom?

102.

In his teachings, the Buddha offers us a way out of our suffering. He teaches that human beings cling to mental positions that trap them in a cycle of suffering. He then teaches that no matter how long we have been stuck in a point of view that causes us to suffer, we can get unstuck. The Buddha uses a particular word for how we get unstuck. He says we *abandon* clinging to the perspectives that have trapped us in suffering.

To abandon a car, we stop. We turn off the engine. Get out of the car. Throw the keys into a nearby river. Then turn and walk away. We do not look back. This was my first success on the road to living honestly. I abandoned the need to be comfortable. I chose growth instead.

Reflection

Choosing growth over comfort is a process that requires momentum. Who is helping you to gain momentum?

103.

I got sober within a close-knit community. Everybody knew when I went to rehab. Everybody knew when I got back. There was no hiding what I was. At two months sober I had to live with the fact that everyone I came into contact with all day, every day, knew I was sick in a way that was not remotely socially acceptable. I had lived for years with the social cachet of being a military cadet and later an officer. But then I began living with a stigma. This gave me a chance to look clear-eyed at the importance I gave to what people thought of me.

It helped that I felt better each day I was sober. It helped that I could feel myself living into something extremely positive. It did not help how precarious it all felt. At two months sober, I knew that however good my foundation was, the odds were still in favor of my drinking myself to death. Faced with this mix of hope and fear, I decided that I did not have time to worry about what other people thought. Caught in a fight for my life, I decided to abandon a specific concern. Caught in a fight for my life, I abandoned caring what other people thought about my fight for my life.

Reflection

There was a great saying going around when I first got sober: "Don't try to do this gracefully." It spoke to the need to put first things first. Just don't drink means just don't die. Are we really going to give someone a vote on how we are not dying one day at a time?

104.

After the initial shock of getting sober began to wear off, it was time to start actually working on my own behalf. Much of what I needed to do during my first year of sobriety was summed up by the phrase "learn and apply." It was my job to learn and apply the principles and practices laid out in my 12-step program. Within that larger framework, there was the specific task of getting honest.

Making meetings a priority was a form of honesty. Showing up to meetings was another. Once the meetings started, there would be a moment when everyone in the room had a chance to introduce themselves. I learned to say, "Hi, my name is Rolf. I'm alcoholic," or simply, "Rolf, alcoholic." I don't know why that phrase stuck, but it was another way I was learning to be honest. When it was my turn, I stated plainly in words that were unambiguous that I was an alcoholic. I would not hedge. I would not explain. I would not qualify. I stated plainly for the record that I met the criteria laid out by Bill Wilson. I was telling my community that I was powerless over alcohol and that my life was unmanageable. Day by day, one ordinary moment at a time, I learned to tell the truth.

Reflection

How and in what way are you learning to tell the truth?

105.

A 12-step meeting is a place where people learn the skills of 12-step sobriety. Much of this learning happens the way it does on a meditation retreat. You just sit quietly, observing. Sometimes the truth comes to you from the speakers in the room. Sometimes the truth comes to you in the form of insight arising within you as you understand something you have spent your whole life not understanding. At a 12-step meeting, there are no designated teachers. The group is the teacher, the group's experience is the teaching. This puts an onus on each member of the group to contribute in a credible fashion to the day's teaching. To make this contribution, the individual member must make a simple yet profound decision. She must decide to be honest.

Sharing honestly about your experience helps everyone in the room reflect on the nature of addiction and skills they are learning in meetings. Sharing honestly about your experiences with a group of recovering people provides you with a chance to integrate what you are learning about living sober in a way that you could not otherwise. The benefit of this honesty is as incalculable to you as it is to the other members of the group. It is the difference between living and dying. It is possible because people are being honest with one another.

Reflection

Are you spending time with other people talking honestly about recovery from addiction? If you are, what is it like? If you are not, what is it like?

106.

After a few days of going to meetings, it was time for me to start speaking about my own experiences. I do not know what I said in those early months, but I remember what it felt like. I would be scared before I spoke—not of the public speaking part but of the enormousness of what I was doing. Speaking in a meeting moves the process forward. When you speak at a meeting, you own the fact of your addiction. When you speak at a meeting, you own the fact of your recovery. I would feel the magnitude of this before I spoke; it made me somewhat breathless. I was scared of the intensity, but I was committed to availing myself of the possibility of sobriety.

When I spoke, I would make every effort to speak honestly about my experience of addiction and recovery. When it was over I would feel I had changed my relationship to recovery *and* my relationship to the group. My willingness to be honest was building a bridge to sobriety. This same bridge took me from the isolation of active addiction to an ever-deepening connection to my sober community.

Reflection

Speaking honestly from a place of compassion builds bridges between people. How was life for you before the bridge was built? How was it afterward?

107.

I had been going to 12-step meetings for several years by the time I began attending workshops at the Kripalu Center for Yoga and Health in Lenox, Massachusetts. Kripalu is a yoga community that has the benefit of communal living, eating, and practice; you are surrounded by your yoga community 24 hours a day. This togetherness becomes a sanctuary in which you can develop far more intimacy with your inner life than you can amidst the hustle and bustle of everyday life. To balance the inward nature of yoga practice, Kripalu offers a *satsang* each evening after dinner in its main hall. The word *satsang* means to sit in the presence of the truth. It also means to dwell in the presence of true people, people who are committed to the truth.

A *satsang* is time set aside for people to get together with the intention of dwelling in the presence of the truth. One night, a teacher might speak. The next night, a musician might play. After a day listening inwardly for the truth, you are able to relax and receive the truth. Your community will do the heavy lifting. You just show up. Taking a seat on my first night, I felt right at home. My 12-step work had formed a bridge back to life. As the years went by, I used that same bridge to find yoga and meditation.

Reflection

What is it like to sit in the presence of the truth? How big a role does time spent in the presence of truth play in your life?

108.

During my first years of yoga practice, it was common for people to greet me or to say farewell with the Sanskrit term *jai bhagwan*. I had no idea what it meant and was too afraid of looking foolish to ask anyone. I would just nod politely, moving on as soon as possible. I attended an evening gathering at the end of which the presenter finished with a series of *jai bhagwans* and then in English said, "Victory, victory, victory to our spirits!" I was moved. What my well-meaning friends had been saying to me was "Victory to your spirit."

I could not believe the resonance of this phrase, how it captured what I had witnessed in 12-step meetings: the victory of the spirit. What better way was there to describe an addict choosing to live sober? That evening in the soft glow of the meditation hall, I was living what it means for the spirit to be victorious.

Reflection

Describe a victory of your spirit. How did it feel?

Before I learned to slow my life down enough to make good choices, I had to slow down my breath enough to feel it. Sobriety brought me into the practice of living honestly. Living honestly got me in touch with the tremendous amount of tension I carried in my body. I was wound up physically, mentally, emotionally. Newly sober, I charged through life, moving from intense perfectionism to white-hot rage and back to intense perfectionism. If I met an attractive woman, I wanted to marry her. If I tried some new activity, I wanted to be the best at it—the best in world! No wonder I had liked a few brewskis. The alternative was manic proving with a side order of shame and a self-doubt salad.

Living honestly allowed me to recognize the benefits of yoga. Breathing mindfully, moving mindfully, and holding poses mindfully allowed me access to a quality of calm awareness I had previously only hoped for. It took about five years for me to work a lifetime of stress out of my body, but I did it, and it has never come back. The first step was getting honest about how I was being in a pose.

Reflection

Just being able to recognize the amount of stress we carry in our bodies is a gift of sobriety. Unless we acknowledge this tension, we eat over it, rage over it, get depressed over it, have sex over it. Are you done with being stressed? What are you willing to do about it?

110.

In my residential work with traumatized children, the term "unresolved issue" came up daily. We called these U.R.I.'s. They were always pressing; as soon as one was resolved, another one arose seemingly out of thin air. Working with these children made us sensitive to the need to address U.R.I.'s head-on in a way that offered real closure. When a child transgressed, she was given the chance to own her behavior, process it, make restitution to the community, then move on. The moving on part was done in the presence of the entire community. Each member of the community contributed to the process of letting something go. When we let something go, we get to begin again.

Getting honest on a yoga mat allowed me to recognize that my entire past was stuck in my young body, making it much older than it was chronologically. Working my way through my first intense yoga training, I encountered 100 ways to be uncomfortable. Each new discomfort in my body was an unresolved issue that I would lament, try to avoid, then meet in a direct way that offered real closure. The first step on the path to freedom was getting honest about how I was being in the pose.

Reflection

Letting go happens mentally, emotionally, energetically, physically. Yoga teaches us how to let go without leaving the pose. What is it like to let go without leaving?

111.

There is a haunting scene in the musical *Hamilton* about parents coping with the death of their child. Two people walking down the street, living in the presence of the unimaginable. Before I started drinking, I had learned to live with the unimaginable. In my world there was no room for me—no safety, no future, no dignity—just survival. Once I got sober, I knew I had a whopping drinking problem, but what I did not know for some time was that the size of my drinking problem reflected the size of my trauma. Once I was sober, I had to accept the degree to which my childhood had left its mark on me. I was what life had made me, which is to say that I was not really me yet.

Stepping onto a yoga mat was like looking into a mirror that shows you all of the choices you have made—how you were strong, when you were afraid, how you loved, how you lost, when you lied, when you did not. The truth comes to you in sensations. We breathe into this part of ourselves to feel our sorrow. We soften to find our wisdom, lengthen to feel our courage, turn to remember, let go to forgive. Our story is told in arcs of sensation, the way fireflies tell an ancient tale with arcs of light across a nighttime sky. A process set in motion by the willingness to be honest.

Reflection

Slow your breathing down enough to be able to feel it. Notice the fireflies stirring, then taking flight, each one a part of how we remember what has always been.

112.

To get sober we have to let go of the false in order to embrace what is true. The process on a yoga mat is the same. As an athlete stepping onto my yoga mat for the first time, I felt I had something to prove. When I was told to do a pose, I attempted to demonstrate my capability. Proving that you are able to do something implies that there is nothing left to learn. At the beginning of my learning process, I acted as if there was nothing left to learn. I did not do this because I thought it was a good idea. I did it because it was all I knew. In order to learn, I had to let go of what I knew. I had to let go of self-protection. I had spent my entire life protecting a child no one else would. To get any further, I would have to let this child out of my protection. It was as hard as it sounds, but it was possible because I was with others who were doing the same.

I could not begin being vulnerable in clear view of my teachers or the other students. It was at the quiet moments at the end of class. When the lights were low, I would lie quietly out of view under a blanket. In the privacy of the *savasana* pose, I would begin to let go. I would feel how twisted and tight my body was against the floor, I would meet this pain with compassion. Breathing gently, I would let my body soften a little, then a little more.

Reflection

We can protect ourselves or we can grow, but we cannot do both at the same time. What does that mean to you today?

113.

I began letting go on my mat. It was glorious. I could not let go in any global or scientific way, but I could feel tension, and I could let go. I could feel the difference it made. I had carried everything life had placed anywhere near me in an ever-expanding sack, the weight of which could be felt in every cell of my body. Being able to let go of something meant the world to me. I felt the immediate impact, relief, and hope. Feeling into my body, noticing where I was holding tension to no purpose, then releasing that tension back into life opened me to a possibility I had never imagined.

My grandmother died holding on to everything. My sister died holding on to everything. My best friend died holding on to everything. My uncles died holding on to everything. But I will not. I still do not know how much I can let go of or how much freedom I can let into my life, but I know how to let go. Each day that I practice, I learn to let go a little more. I will not die having never known the feeling of freedom.

Reflection

What does freedom mean to you? How does it feel?

114.

There is a barn on a hill in western Massachusetts. On Sunday mornings during the warm months, a 12-step meeting is held there. To get there, you have to drive along a narrow dirt road that winds through a forest up a small hill. The road is bordered by stone walls built the way farmers built them hundreds of years ago. You park in the dusty farmyard or in the grass by the side of the road. The seats at the meeting are a hodgepodge of metal fold-ups and wooden chairs that might have come from someone's study. These are placed on the grass, so they feel a little tippy, but the view makes up for it. The smell is a blend of grass, trees, and earth. A blue summer sky is dotted with soft clouds. Sitting, we read the preamble of the program, which states how we understand addiction, how we get well, what we intend to do about it. We share a moment of silence, then begin the healing process called telling the truth.

Reflection

Where do you go to be in the presence of the truth? How do you tell your truth?

115.

I started attending meditation retreats in an effort to feel better. One of the popular phrases of that time was "I am overwhelmed." It could mean "I am involved in a lot of important stuff, so don't expect the same amount of accountability that you would expect from a less important friend." It could also mean "Pity me and do not hold me accountable the way you would any other adult in your life." It could also mean "Don't blame me for poor performance right now; no one in my position could possibly excel, and I'll be awesome later when I am less overwhelmed." I went to my first meditation retreat because I was "overwhelmed," but no one was really buying it. I felt I needed a break. I was not even aware that there was a connection between meditating and getting honest. I thought it was all about the stillness, the days without the hassle of being overwhelmed.

The form of the retreat I ended up at was unremittingly intense. There were 45-minute seated meditations all day long. Our breaks were 45-minute walking meditations. It was overwhelming. I was with myself in silence all day long while I attempted something I found very difficult. It was revealing. I saw what was going to work. I saw what wasn't. I saw what was true about myself as I went through something difficult. Back home, I looked at the people in my life. Every person I met was going through something difficult. The difference between me and most of the people I observed was that I had been given the chance to live a difficult life with a little more awareness, a little more understanding, a little more truth. This difference meant that I was beginning to meet pain with compassion, suffering with understanding.

Reflection

How does it feel when you are able to meet pain with compassion, suffering with understanding?

116.

The reason I felt overwhelmed in my life was that I felt like a failure in many ways. I had the outward appearance of success, but I was not as good a husband as I wanted to be. I was not as good a father as I wanted to be. I was nowhere near as good a friend as I wanted to be, or son, or brother. The only thing I did well was teach yoga, which made me more uncomfortable with myself because of the pedestal my students put me on. Everything I attempted felt tainted by a form of self-interest that manifested itself in extremely shortsighted behavior. I simply could not get out of my own way.

Sitting day after day alone with myself, I followed the instructions I received from my teachers. This precipitated an inventory process in which I observed the ways that I judged myself, the ways that I simply could not accept myself as I was. It was a hard, sad process. I learned from my teachers that before I could understand something, I had to be willing to stand under it. This could not have been more the case than when it came to the harsh judgment I was placing upon myself. I sat with it, felt the weight of it, felt the ouch of it. I felt the truth of it. I was not being fair with myself at all. This was the beginning of understanding.

Reflection

To understand something we must be willing to stand under it. To stand under something difficult, we must have support. Do you have the support you need to stand under the big lessons of your recovery?

117.

To see how I was treating myself was a game changer because it made me look at my relationship to the truth in general. Sitting day after day with the half-baked judgments I was leveling at myself forced me to consider that I appeared to be indifferent to the truth. It was enough for me to have an opinion. The opinion did not have to be supported by facts in any way; it simply needed to reflect my point of view, which was just a lot of opinions I had had for a while. This was pretty shabby. As I unpacked my relationship to myself, I saw how unexamined it was, how uninformed. How the truth was like a professional no one bothered to consult before embarking on a perilous journey.

Wisdom and compassion are two sides of a coin. The coin is truth; when truth is present, they are too. The truth worked its way into the soil of my self-hate, bringing the light of wisdom. The truth worked its way into the soil of my self-hate, bringing the gentle regard of my heart. To look truthfully is to look with understanding, to look with kindness, to look with compassion. In the light of my own understanding I could see how I caused suffering with ignorance and delusion. I saw how I did it. I saw how we all do it. Like an astronaut is forever changed when she looks down on our planet, I was changed when I saw what we do to ourselves.

Reflection

It is an article of faith in yoga that we are all fighting a hard battle. Can you look truthfully at your own hard battle? How does that change your understanding of the people in your life?

118.

As a child I had kept my sadness secret. I had felt alone, utterly unwelcome. I was a black child. There was no place for me. This filled me with shame. I hid it behind everything I said and did. My greatest fear was the truth. Lies were my only protection against the shame I felt. With lies, I could be someone else.

Getting sober was my first experience with the nobility of honesty. I had been honest as a military officer to avoid consequences. In sobriety, I practiced honesty to step into a new life. As years went by, I found I did not need my protective layer of lies. It was a process. I would be honest about my drinking but not about my fears or desires. I would be honest at work or in meetings but not with my friends or family. I would be honest at work, at meetings, with friends, with family, but not with myself. Sitting quietly, doing nothing, day after day on meditation retreats, I began to get honest with myself. Sitting quietly, doing nothing, I began to let go of the desire to be someone else.

Reflection

What is the relationship between getting sober and no longer wanting to be someone else?

Truth

Our relationship with the truth determines the success we will experience in any given moment, with any given spiritual practice, on any given path to sobriety. To close this chapter, I wanted to devote a few essays to each of our three traditions to make the case for the importance of honesty and how we should practice it.

119.

When I think of the role of truth on the path to freedom, I think of the need to know that I have given it my best. How do you know that you have done all that you can? What is an honest effort? The Yoga Sutras are a window into the lives of countless people who have asked the same question. They present us with a short list of habits to put us in the right place, doing the right thing for the right reasons. These are the habits of discipline, self-study, and proper orientation. Our yoga elders believed that when these factors are in place, you are doing all that you can, with all that you have, in the place where you are.

Instead of identifying a singular quality to embrace, yoga offers us three that we must bring into harmony: discipline, self-study, and orientation. Discipline in this sense is energetic effort, self-study provides us with a sense of what we are working on, and orientation toward the ideal keeps our eyes on the prize. The world of the yoga elders was very different from ours, but their challenge was much the same. They were human beings trying to give life an honest effort. Their solution was to bring energy and enthusiasm to the process of self-study in the service of freedom.

Reflection

Bring energy and enthusiasm to the process of self-study in the service of freedom. How is this happening for you? What is helping you do this one day at a time?

120.

Discipline is a word that most addicts have trouble with. I wrote "Disciplinary action" under my senior yearbook photo as my pet peeve. Discipline was not my friend. Discipline was a form of social control. I did not know who I was or what I wanted, so how could anyone else? Yoga rebranded the concept for me. My teachers said that we are free to choose the disciplines to which we bind ourselves. We are free to choose. These disciplines create and maintain our freedom. We are free to choose to bind ourselves to disciplines that make our lives work.

This sounded about right. Binding myself to the discipline of sobriety had created and maintained my freedom. Binding myself to the discipline of a 12-step program had created and maintained a number of new freedoms in my life. I saw how my life was demonstrating the relationship between discipline and freedom.

Reflection

What disciplines are creating freedom in your life today?

121.

According to the core teachings of yoga, we are free to bind ourselves to disciplines that create and maintain our freedom. This is a paradox. We are already free, but we need disciplines to maintain our freedom. Is this true? It was for me. I kept it simple. I am alive, and I have to eat to stay alive. Being alive is a process; freedom is a process. We live in a world that is permanently impermanent. Everything around us is in a constant state of transformation, arising-changing-passing-arising-changing-passing. Why would freedom be any different? Do freedoms stick around without some sort of maintenance? My experience hasn't been as such. I have had to choose my freedom over and over again by binding myself to behaviors that maintain my freedom. Cultivating the habit of discipline is cultivating the possibility of freedom.

There is another takeaway from the habit of discipline: self-respect. When I follow through on a commitment, however small, I experience a measure of self-respect. *Follow-through* was not exactly the word that came to people's minds when they thought of me during my drinking. Living several miles from follow-through was a lame place to be; people around me got to be the follow-through friend, the follow-through colleague. I did not. Putting sober days together is an act of follow-through. As the days added up, the follow-through started to show up in other areas of my life. I could be counted on to show up to work on time, dressed appropriately, with a good attitude. I started to see myself as that guy, the one who could be counted on to show up. The discipline of sobriety had given me an energy and enthusiasm for discipline in life.

Reflection

In sobriety, we learn to let follow-through happen one day at a time. What are you following through on these days?

122.

My teachers taught me that disciplines create and maintain our freedom. They also taught me that a discipline is a net positive behavior. We get more energy out of a discipline than we put into it. As this dynamic gains traction in our life, we start to have all the energy and enthusiasm we need to meet the challenges life brings.

As I write this, there is a young man making history named Kyle Snyder. Still in college, he has won three straight world wrestling titles, including an Olympic gold medal. Recently he beat the best wrestler in the world to gain his third world title. By winning this match, he also secured the world team title for the United States for the first time since 1995. He knew this match was coming for months. The night he walked out to meet his fate, everything rested on his very young shoulders, but his focus was not on the burden; his focus was on the opportunity. He was profoundly excited to be in *this* place meeting *this* challenge because he had done the work. He had done the work for many years. He had developed momentum in his life. He smiles when he talks of things that would make almost anyone else uncertain or afraid. His discipline has given him a profound passion for the life he has chosen.

Reflection

Our disciplines create and maintain our freedom. The experience turns habits into passions. Are you beginning to develop a passion for sobriety?

123.

Self-study is the process of learning and applying spiritual teachings. The habit of discipline cultivates energy; the habit of self-study cultivates skill. The skills of yoga are not simply studied; they are lived. They require all the energy discipline can deliver.

Learning in yoga looks a lot like learning in a 12-step program. There is literature to read, peers to chat with, mentors to listen to. Yoga excels in creating the space between learning and living called practice. Yoga poses, Yogic breathing exercises, and meditation combine to offer a student a place to practice a skill before bringing it into daily life. The separation is not completely distinct, though. You can "get" something just by hearing it said by a teacher. You can believe you have no idea what a teacher is saying, only for it to land while you are on your mat or cushion. You can half learn it on your cushion, only for it to make full sense once you are walking your dog. Yoga has created an extremely dynamic learning process by creating a form of experiential education that constitutes a bridge between the classroom and everyday life. Self-study turns the formal study of yoga theory, the experiential education of practice, and the mechanics of everyday life into a congruent learning process. The aim of this process is an honest effort at living your yoga.

Reflection

It is hard to learn and apply more than one new life skill at a time. If you had to name one life skill you are learning to apply these days, what would it be?

124.

When I teach yoga, I explain to students that a yoga class is where we practice the skills of yoga. At the beginning of the process, I spend a period of time defining the skill we will be practicing, just as a science teacher will spend time at the chalkboard before she takes her students into the laboratory for the actual experiment. The "dharma talk" is the time at the chalkboard, the "yoga class" is the time spent in the laboratory experimenting with the "chemicals" of sensation.

A principle I often teach is that when we connect to the present moment, the mind becomes still. I state this to my students before class, then briefly review how they will be connecting to the present moment through the quality of effort they bring to their poses. The students then spend the remainder of class moving from pose to pose, balancing effort with ease in their bodies. Each time they do so, they see what happens to the mind. The hypothesis is that as the body "finds the middle between effort and ease," the mind finds the moment. The students conduct this experiment over and over again during class so that they leave the class familiar with the experience of the mind resting in the moment. They have taken a principle off the page and into their felt experience in class so they can then conduct this same experiment throughout the day.

Reflection

The three stages of learning are:

1. *Defining terms*
2. *Applying lessons in a "laboratory" setting*
3. *Applying lessons in everyday life*

How do these three stages show up in the spiritual education that exists in your life right now?

125.

Proper orientation in the 12-step program is articulated in the preamble of Alcoholics Anonymous as "the desire to stop drinking." Everything one does in the program is oriented toward the achievement of "contented sobriety." Proper orientation in yoga is defined as resting in a form of awareness that contains neither attachment nor aversion. Everything one does in yoga is oriented toward the achievement of non-attached involvement with life. Proper orientation gives us a means to evaluate the functionality of a choice or practice. In other words, it helps us answer the question "Does this choice move me toward my goal? Is there wisdom here?" Meditation teachers use the phrase "onward-leading" to describe a choice that has proper orientation.

Just as 12-step programs possess a singleness of purpose, yoga's proper orientation lends a pragmatic focus to its practices. The measure is not in days sober but in the quality of our relationship to the moment. Am I learning to connect and rest in connection? Is the way I am spending my days creating more or less attachment, more or less aversion? Am I learning to rest in the space between wanting and not wanting? Can I bring this form of awareness into my work, my friendships, my family? What helps?

Reflection

How intense is your hour-to-hour experience of wanting or not wanting? What cools this? What heats it up?

126.

I bring proper orientation into the classes I teach with the phrase "resting in connection." Resting in connection means letting go of wanting anything from that connection. In proper orientation we are in a pure form of awareness that does not include attachment or aversion. Although this is the ultimate goal of yoga, the ordinary yoga student can achieve this type of connection often and easily. The trick is in how we approach the challenge. If we approach it as "pure awareness," we will wonder what pure awareness means. If we approach it as listening to the wind through trees, we will just listen without attachment or aversion. After listening for a while, we will feel the breath, and then we will move smoothly. As this is happening, we will learn to reflect on our experience. What is it like to breathe, to move smoothly? What is it like to feel? Later we won't do anything at all, becoming still by allowing stillness to happen. What is it like to allow?

Once I teach the direct experience, the next challenge is getting students to understand what just happened so they can move back into this form of connection without the support of the class. If I describe yoga in terms of exalted states, students show up alienated from the proper orientation of their practice. They just come for the workout or for stress reduction because they do not feel included in the actual intention of the practice. The trick has been for students to realize that every time they really want to connect to a smell, taste, or sensation, they do. Which is to say, every time they have proper orientation, they will succeed.

Reflection

What is your experience when you move from thinking to just feeling? Just tasting? Just listening? What is your experience when you incline the mind toward the present moment?

127.

Cael Sanderson, the coach of my favorite college wrestling team, teaches his athletes that they cannot control the results but they can control the effort they put into their training; they can control the effort they put into every position in competition. He teaches his kids to do all they can, with all that they have, in the place where they are. Yoga breaks this down for us by giving us three pursuits that, taken together, amount to an honest effort.

1. Discipline: We are what we habitually do.

2. Self-study: If we know better, we will do better.

3. Proper orientation: You hit what you aim at.

A circle is formed by aiming, doing, and learning.

Reflection

What are you aiming at? How is that expressed by what you habitually do? What is it like to learn about life this way?

128.

While yoga defines an honest effort in terms of discipline, self-study, and proper orientation, 12-step programs have described the essentials of recovery as honesty, open-mindedness, and willingness. This H.O.W. of a 12-step program teaches recovering people to be responsible for how they are relating to the learning process of living sober. In this approach to freedom, an honest effort begins not so much with what you are doing but with how you are being.

It is no small irony that I find myself writing this. For years I have taught that "the pose is what you are doing, yoga is how you are being in the pose." And in this particular instance, the Eastern woo-woo yoga take is more about the doing, while in the West, the somewhat religious 12-step program is all about the being. Kudos to life for its ability to keep serving up the surprises! That being said, the 12-step programs are making a very real contribution to this discussion. They are saying that you may not be able to control the circumstances in which you find yourself, but you can control whether or not you are being honest, open-minded, and willing.

Reflection

Recovery offered me ways to channel my energy that were both humble and visionary. I could be waiting tables in a shabby restaurant while applying ancient teachings that cut to the heart of the human condition. Can you feel the visionary quality of honesty, open-mindedness, and willingness as an approach to your future?

129.

Being honest in recovery begins with how we talk about our addiction. We learn to be honest with the right people at the right time in order to get the help that we need. We learn to work wisely with the discomfort that comes with the vulnerability of honesty. It sucks to be vulnerable in this way at this time in our lives when we feel so low, but the cost-benefit analysis is strongly in favor of taking the hit and getting honest. We can endure the pain of getting clean, or we can endure the pain of an addict's death. There's no real choice here.

This form of honesty is more than enough. It addresses the life-or-death crossroads that every addict faces. If we want a life worth getting sober for, we have to learn to broaden the circle of our honesty to include the rest of what we think, say, and do. The honesty of a successful recovery is self-honesty. Twelve-step programs teach us to bring our attention to how we are relating to a situation. They teach us to feel the difference between honesty and rationalization. Then, miraculously, they teach the habit of choosing honesty.

Reflection

A successful support group for recovery from addiction helps us choose self-honesty in a way that feels fun and life-affirming. Have you found that support?

130.

My meditation teachers have helped me look at the near cause of something. What happens right before I do something self-destructive? What happens right before I make a good choice? What keeps me in what Bill Wilson called the bondage of self? What helps me be free? The concept of near cause helps us to see how things connect, how we can put a series of positive events in motion the same way we have put a series of negative events in motion. The practice of self-honesty is what happens right before we become open-minded. Open-mindedness makes us teachable. Considering the fact that we are learning a new way of life, this chain of events is worthy of investigation.

While sitting in a meeting or on my meditation cushion, reflecting on my mind instead of reacting to it, I cannot escape a few pertinent facts.

1. I am often ignorant of critical information.

2. I am often delusional with regard to point number one (i.e., I do not know that I do not know).

3. I often wish I could do better, but I just don't know how.

When I reflect on my mind instead of reacting to it, I am able to see that it has been closed to information that would have protected me from harm. This hurts, but it gives me hope. What will change next time if my mind is open?

Reflection

When we bring honesty and open-mindedness together, we create a teachable moment called humility. Can you feel the difference between humility and humiliation?

131.

When we combine honesty and open-mindedness, we find our-selves on sacred ground, the place where the learning of a lifetime can happen. There is a form of courage that we must possess if we are to become an explorer in this new world. It is called humility. Humility is to have the courage to say, "I do not know, but I would like to learn." It is a breeze that sweeps away the fog. It is a heart quality; it is a state of mind; it is a virtue. Humility is the cause, and willingness is the effect. Humility opens the door, but willing-ness allows us to take the first step.

Reflection

Sobriety is equal parts humility and willingness. Describe how you have found these qualities of heart and mind when you needed them. How have they saved your life?

132.

As an active addict, I wanted things very badly. I fought for them. Sometimes I earned them. When the dust settled, whatever the outcome, I was robbed of the good that could have come from my efforts because I did not know if I had done my best. Sometimes I knew that I had shown courage or intelligence or skill, but there was still the unanswered question: Was this the best I could have done? Because of this inability to know something so critical about the challenges I set before myself, I could not move on. I could not learn my lessons; I could not grow.

During my first year of sobriety, I became a waiter. It was a humble job that turned out to be harder than it looked. I was working at a restaurant that had already declared bankruptcy, and my manager was a very active addict. Things often went wrong. I made mistakes. There were days that I left with an extremely bruised ego, but there were never days when I did not know if I had done my best.

During my short time in sobriety, I had already learned how to give something my all. The job paid poorly. It had no future. But I was at peace with my part in it. I became proud of the lessons I learned in that dim, dirty restaurant. I was proud of the honesty, the open-mindedness, the willingness it took to learn those lessons. I have been able to build on them. I have been able to grow from them.

Reflection

We can learn our lessons and then walk on if we have done our best. Closure is possible. An honest effort prepares us for the next challenge. Are you giving yourself the steady foundation of an honest effort so that you can reach for your next level?

133.

Yoga has given us specific practices for learning discipline, self-study, and proper orientation; from yoga we learn what to *do*. From 12-step programs we are given a way to *be*: honest, open-minded, willing. Meditation teachers offer us three stages for *how* to learn: by hearing, then seeing, then being. As a student, I was instructed to become adept at hearing what was taught, to become a good listener, to ask questions. Then to see if what was being taught was true, to see it for myself, without taking someone else's word for it, to see if it was true in my own experience and in the world around me. Finally, I learned that if a teaching proves to be true, be it.

The Buddha taught that once you know something to be true, you must embody it. Having made an honest effort in the learning process, make an honest effort at living what you have learned.

Reflection

This final section, on truth, has laid out a number of ways to make an honest effort. This type of effort is directed at learning a new way of life. What are you hearing, seeing, and being these days that feels new in the best possible way?

134.

As a traumatized young person, I simply could not rest in connection long enough to form a relationship to the truth of anything. I couldn't really learn in school, I couldn't really connect in my friendships, I couldn't really be a part of my family. I was there and I was not. Before meditation, the closest I came to resting in connection was when things were intense. Sports were intense, sex was intense, drugs were intense, getting very drunk was intense. Intensity could hold me for a while, but it could not make me whole.

The intensity of getting sober held my attention too. As I lived through a life-and-death struggle, the meetings felt like the greatest show on earth. People fighting for their lives is intense. I listened closely. I learned to listen. Then my meditation teachers offered me a way to bring my meditation practice into my listening. They taught that I should stay in my body while I listened . . . stay connected to how I was breathing while I listened . . . stay connected to how I was sitting while I listened. *When you are sitting, know that you are sitting. When you are breathing, know that you are breathing.* Bring awareness to how you are listening to what is being taught. Are you listening with attachment or aversion? Are you simply resting in listening? What is listening like?

Reflection

Begin to include yourself in your listening. Is there attachment or aversion present? What is your listening like?

135.

As I began to include my felt experience in my understanding of the act of listening, I was able to watch my reaction to what I was listening to. Was there a mental reaction, an emotional reaction, a physical reaction, all of the above, or none of the above? I became able to watch how I was learning. Was there a steady connection to the process, or was I drifting in and out? Did a reaction pull me into a drama that was distracting me? What pulled me into a reaction? What made me drift? When was I asking a question because I really wanted to learn something? When was I asking a question to prove something or to assert control over a process that I had an aversion to?

Listening in this way set the stage for the moment when I learned something new. I would be calmly applying myself to the process of listening mindfully, and then there it would be. You never know when you are going to hear something new, even something that will change your life. All you can do is become as adept as possible at listening. Doing the work of listening makes us sensitive to what is happening right now. Sometimes what is happening is a concept slowly coming into focus. Sometimes what is happening is a new world dancing out onto the stage to take a bow. Sometimes what is happening is genuine insight.

Reflection

Recovery is a learning process. The first step in that process is listening. For recovery to flourish, we must become passionate listeners. Can you make it your business to become a passionate listener?

136.

Once we have learned something new—a teaching, a principle, a practice—we are instructed to see for ourselves whether or not it is true, useful, or onward-leading. This process may take days, months, or years. It does not really matter how long it takes because this kind of information lands only when we are ready. There is no pushing this river. So with the pressure off, we have to live into the question until we have found ourselves living into the answer.

The first level of this inquiry is whether or not something is true in your own experience. If I do this practice, will it help me stay sober? Will it help me rest in connection with the present moment? Is there wisdom here? The next level is whether or not something holds true in the world around us. When I got sober, I already knew violence was the worst possible outcome in my personal life, but I did not know if it was true in the world. Does war make things better or worse? Every day of my life I have lived with people killing each other somewhere on earth; it is a painful truth of my existence. Reflecting on this awful truth, I can honestly say it has never made anything better. Once we know something is true, we must embody it.

Reflection

We are given two levels of inquiry: Is it true in my life? Is it true in the world around me? Once we know something to be true, we must embody it. What new truth are you embodying?

137.

In 1939, Bill Wilson encouraged his fellow addicts to "be the dharma" when he wrote down the final step of the 12-step program he pioneered: "Having had a spiritual awakening as a result of these steps, we tried to carry this message to alcoholics, and to practice these principles in all our affairs."

The elements of an honest effort are:

1. Be honest.

2. Be open-minded.

3. Be willing.

4. Learn to listen.

5. Learn to know the truth.

6. Learn to live the truth.

7. Study spiritual disciplines.

8. Practice a discipline until it becomes a passion.

9. Keep first things first.

Reflection

Make your own list.

Chapter Four

Action

The poet Rumi wrote, "Let the beauty that you love be what you do." In this chapter, we will be looking at how we close the gap between our values and our actions.

138.

The Buddha sat in meditation in an effort to understand himself. He saw that certain actions led to suffering. He saw that others led to well-being. To make things easier on his students, he taught them general rules or precepts to help them organize their daily lives. He called living according to these precepts "wise action." It was not enough for his students to merely follow his instructions. He taught them to observe cause and effect in order to see what was true about a given behavior. When I do something, does it lead to freedom or suffering? Does it lead to harmony or discord? Every action taken wisely would not waste any energy on the costly consequences of unskillful behavior. Every action taken wisely has the benefit of being onward-leading. Every action taken wisely moves you closer to freedom further from suffering.

Reflection

Consider the elegance of wise action: zero negative consequences and maximal positive benefits. Not good or bad. Not sin or redemption. Just wise. How has wise action shown up in your life since you got clean or sober?

139.

The precepts taught by the Buddha are common sense if your goal is well-being. This common sense can also be seen in the underpinnings of yoga and the 12-step approach to living usefully. The Buddha taught his precepts as vows that his students undertook. The word *undertake*—to take on or make a beginning—speaks to how learning to live skillfully is a process. The vows are:

1. I undertake the training rule to abstain from killing.

2. I undertake the training rule to abstain from taking that which is not freely given.

3. I undertake the training rule to avoid sexual misconduct.

4. I undertake the training rule to abstain from false speech.

5. I undertake the training rule to abstain from the use of intoxicants.

At the beginning of a meditation retreat, we take these vows. The vows give the students permission to focus on the work they are there to do. They give permission for the students to trust that the people around them will conduct themselves in a way that supports their work. Over time, I have grown to love being in a community that has abandoned harmful behavior in any form so that we can do the work that we came to do.

Reflection

When we get sober, we undertake a life of non-harming. We begin by refraining from the use of intoxicants. We come to see that this been a form of harm that we have done to ourselves. Over time, we broaden the circle of our non-harming. What are you including these days?

140.

A friend gave me a yoga mat more than 15 years ago. It is a great mat, the only one I have ever used since then. I got a block to match it. Another friend gave me the only meditation pillow I have ever had. These are my tools. A mat. A block. A cushion. They have held me through it all. Last year I taught at a retreat at my meditation center. At the end of the retreat, I signed books. After that, there was a lot of handshaking, hugging, and goodbyes. When I rushed to my ride home, I had my suitcase but left my mat, block, and cushion behind. It would be almost a year before I would return. My wife was alarmed. She asked me if there was something we could do. I said no and that I would get them when I went back. A year later, at the beginning of my next retreat, I went to the closet where the props are kept. I took my belongings down from the shelf, walked to the meditation hall, and put them down. It was time to begin again.

The Dalai Lama says that it is priceless to live without harming. I would add that it is priceless to know that your community has undertaken the training rule of non-harming. I knew that my belongings would be there when I needed them to be, just as I knew that my community would be there when I needed them.

Reflection

The precepts are here so that we can trust enough to let go and do the work. What helps you let go and do the work?

141.

The Buddha sat in meditation in an effort to understand himself. Sitting with the intention of self-awareness, the Buddha noticed that a steady mind was necessary. Sitting in an effort to understand himself, he noticed that a compassionate heart was necessary. These qualities had to be in place if he was to succeed in his task. Sitting day after day with the same intention, he noticed that certain actions disrupted his mind; these same actions troubled his heart. Sitting with a disturbed mind taught him about the nature of a disturbed mind. Sitting with a troubled heart taught him about the nature of a troubled heart. These are skillful insights, but they were not what he was seeking, any more than someone seeking to know the ocean can know it from observing a single wave.

Sitting day after day, he identified the qualities of heart, body, and mind that led to the understanding he sought. The experience of these qualities was calm, clear, kind awareness. Sitting day after day, he identified the actions that made calm, clear, kind awareness impossible. Having understood this, he undertook the training rule to abstain from the actions that made his training impossible.

Reflection

It is important to understand that the spiritual training contained in this book is highly practical. Ethical precepts are included in all three traditions because of the nature of the change we want to make in our lives. Can you see the connection between the change you want and undertaking the training rule to abstain from harming yourself or others?

142.

The first precept the Buddha laid out is the same precept Patanjali, the author of the Yoga Sutras, led with: non-harming. It has been my experience that this is pretty much the only precept; everything else is just window dressing. We are encouraged in all three traditions to undertake the training rule of non-harming when it comes to anything we are involved in. Otherwise we create mental, emotional, physical, financial, sexual, professional, and interpersonal chaos. This is not news to us. We are the pros when it comes to that kind of chaos. The question is whether or not we believe we can, want to, or should do anything about it.

When Bill Wilson described us as children of chaos he wasn't exaggerating. Many of us were brought up in chaos, only to leave home directly into the chaos of our addiction. We have also been agents of chaos—bulls in china shops, tornadoes in the lives of those around us. Over the years we have developed a loyalty to chaos. We tend to be found where chaos abounds. I knew as I went through military training that I was more comfortable in danger and chaos than most people. When we get sober, we have to hang up our chaos spurs in order to join the rest of the human race. It helps that the first rule of sober club is to do no harm. We may have loved chaos, but we love the people in our lives more.

Reflection

Can you feel how sobriety and non-harming are basically the same undertaking?

143.

I was a strong kid who learned rage from my mother. She would work herself into a violent state several times a week. I am not sure if everyone has this sort of rage in them, but living around it, I knew that I could access it if I had to. I never did. I was the strongest kid in my class, which meant I had to defend my class's honor regularly. In the 1970s that meant getting into fistfights. When I wasn't actually fighting, my classmates loved to wrestle. Rambunctiousness was our default setting throughout elementary school. I found myself having to choose not to fight in anger often; I knew that if I went there, the way my mother did, someone would get hurt. I could feel in me the will to destroy, but I refused to destroy another child.

I spent my elementary years hiding my true physical capacity. In middle school, I joined the wrestling team. I would walk out on the mat and fight someone to defend my school's honor, but there were rules. No one was going to get hurt. By undertaking the competition rules of non-harming, I was allowed to do my best. It was during the next 10 years of wrestling that I was able to discover my true physical potential. Unlocking that potential was central to my ability to get sober. Later it became central to my ability to teach yoga.

Reflection

We bind ourselves to disciplines in order reach our full potential the way a tomato plant is bound to a trellis so that it can grow toward the sun. What discipline have you undertaken that has allowed you to grow toward the light?

144.

For the past 20 years I have been spending time at three retreat centers that have undertaken the Buddhist training rule to abstain from killing. A feature of these places is that the surrounding wildlife knows it. In particular, turkey and deer take advantage of our vows. They live on the grounds, free from interference from the mountain lions that lurk in the surrounding hills. At the retreat in upstate New York, things get a little dicey because black bears will wander down to our compost pile without a care in the world. A sea lion jumped into a boat to get away from marauding orcas. In Houston, a hawk got into a cab, refusing to leave, in order to save itself from Hurricane Harvey. In each case, we saved the animal's life.

Animals know something about us that we do not. They feel our potential for kindness. They feel our potential for compassion. When they must, they will call upon that potential. Our fear is not our destiny. Our rage is not our destiny. The animals that share the planet with us already know this. We seem to be the last to know that love is our true nature. When we must, we call upon that potential. If you are reading this, that time has come.

Reflection

How often is your first impulse compassion? Start to notice this impulse.

145.

There is a joy that is present when people in recovery come together. It is not present because of our circumstances or what we have acquired. It is there because we have lucked into the best choice a person can make. For reasons beyond our comprehension, we have been able to arrest a fatal decline. We have been able to see how we have been harming ourselves. We have allowed this information into our hearts. We have considered it deeply. We have undertaken to abstain from harming ourselves. This relieves us of a spiritual toxin that has sickened us in ways too all-encompassing to describe; all we can do is describe what it is like to be without it. Or we can let Bill Wilson do it for us from the *Big Book*:

> We are going to know a new freedom and a new happiness. We will not regret the past nor wish to shut the door on it. We will comprehend the word serenity and we will know peace.

Namaste.

Reflection

We bind ourselves to healthy disciplines in order to create and maintain our freedom.

146.

The Buddha sat in meditation in an effort to understand himself. He noticed four types of effort that led to freedom. One effort was the work of avoiding unskillful mind states. Another was the effort to abandon unskillful mind states once they have arisen. Another was the cultivation of healthy mind states. Yet another was to maintain healthy mind states once they have been cultivated. He saw that one of these forms of effort would always be present. We can either put forth the effort to work with our mind states or we can be swept away by them like a bridge in a flood.

When people in recovery say they are sick and tired of being sick and tired, they are saying that they are weary of being swept up in unskillful mind states. Our drinking, or drugging, or bingeing, or purging, or gambling was a symptom of unskillful mind states that we were trying to manage with our addictions. Once we put down the addiction, we have to deal with difficult mind states. Undertaking a set of ethical precepts is the first step in dealing with our own mind. Having undertaken the vow of non-harming, we become sensitive to the state of our mind. We recognize the relationship between the quality of the mind state and the quality of the behavior. Ultimately we realize that there are four efforts, four responsibilities, that are always present. Avoid the negative, abandon it when it arises, cultivate the good, and maintain the good when it is present.

Reflection

Before we can put forth the effort to address the habits of our mind, we must recognize that they exist. Are you learning to watch your own mind? Are you beginning to see the relationship between your state of mind and the state of your behavior?

Ethical precepts work to prevent the vicious cycle of negative mind states giving rise to negative behaviors that give rise to yet more negative mind states. Precepts address this cycle by encouraging us to abstain from the negative behavior. But like the addict who is no longer using, the Yogi who is abstaining from negative behavior still has to work with negative mind states.

Ethical precepts focus our attention on skillful and unskillful behavior. As we practice a precept, we first bring our awareness to gross acts of misconduct like physical and verbal abuse. Over time we start to see the value in bringing our awareness to the subtle microaggressions that contaminate our relationships. We move from the gross to the subtle. As this movement deepens, we find that we are no longer observing our behavior. We are now learning to observe the mind states that precede a behavior. We start to see a mind state *as* a behavior. This is when the work of the precepts starts to inhabit our inner life.

Reflection

Have you considered your thoughts to be behaviors subject to the same ethical guidelines as your physical actions?

148.

Once you have begun to see that an ethical precept is a commitment to observe a behavior from its inception as a mind state to its midpoint as an action to its conclusion as a consequence, you have begun the inner work of mindfulness in earnest. The Yogis liken this to the work of a gardener. The mind state is the seed, the action is the plant, the consequence is the fruit. The wise gardener puts her attention on the seeds she is planting.

Reflection

Are you willing to look at the seeds you are planting with your thoughts? Can you see the connection between the seed and the fruit?

149.

The Buddha taught us how to grow a garden of well-being. We are instructed to look at our behaviors. Which ones lead to suffering? Which lead to freedom? We are taught to look at our thoughts. Which lead to suffering? Which lead to freedom? We are then given specific instructions in each instance. It is better to deal with an acorn than an oak tree. Watch the mind become adept at avoiding negative mind states. A shift of our attention is easier than making amends. If a negative mind state has arisen, you are already in ill will or greed. Learn to let it go. Run, don't walk, to the nearest exit.

The next two behaviors are easier because they are something to do rather than something to stop. It begins with the cultivation of the opposite. If the problem is ill will, we are to cultivate loving-kindness. We do this primarily with our thoughts. In Buddhism, we spend time in meditation repeating loving statements toward ourselves and others. We practice the habit of thinking kind thoughts. Likewise, in my 12-step program, we are taught to pray for people we resent. This is planting good seeds. Once we are in a state of loving-kindness, we are instructed to learn to rest in this state. We are not grasping it. We are resting in it like someone learning to rest in sensation— the sweet smell of eucalyptus, the pleasant warmth of a bath, the beauty of a sunset. Rest in the sensation of a heart open in kindness. The fruit of this heart-mind state is harmony.

Reflection

The effort put into planting the seeds of well-being can't be used to plant the seeds of suffering. Learn to put a good day together. Learn to spend your days planting the seeds of well-being.

150.

Take one of these forms of effort and practice it.

1. If you don't want a haircut, don't go into a barbershop. Learn to spend your time in places that support your sobriety.

2. If you are in a hole, stop digging. When a mind state or behavior is giving you trouble, leave it like you would a sinking ship.

3. Cultivate positive mind states through affirmation, meditation, and positive habits of speech. Practice being the change you want to see in the world.

4. Enjoy the fruits of your labors. Learn to rest in positive mind states. Learn to see them as your natural state.

When you have practiced one form of effort for a while, include another until all four have become ingrained in your everyday life.

Reflection

Which practices support you in this work? Meetings? Meditation? Exercise? Yoga? What connections are you observing between the various practices?

151.

My meditation teachers taught me that your goal is the mountain that you are climbing. Your intention is the manner in which you take each step. A precept or ethical discipline is the goal. The intention is to unlearn negative mind states that lead to the violation of a precept. The intention is to cultivate positive mind states that make adhering to a precept sustainable.

A simple example of this is the 12-step goal of not drinking. To help make this possible, we are taught to avoid the states of Hungry-Angry-Lonely-Tired, or H.A.L.T. These states are particularly problematic for someone new to the precept of abstaining from intoxicants. A spiritual community can help us by identifying states of mind that don't work, just as it can identify behaviors that don't work. The individual's job is to start with the foundation her community has laid out in terms of goals and intentions, then build from there. The beginning we make using the guidance of our teachers allows us to develop the skills necessary to undertake our own journey.

Reflection

What state of mind helps you stay true to your goals? What state of mind makes it difficult?

152.

The framework of goals and intentions allows us to apply a spiritual principle in our day-to-day existence. The process of learning a principle becomes the process of living it. In the beginning, we are honest, open-minded, and willing as we approach the idea of a spiritual precept. We do our homework so we know how the principle is supposed to be practiced. We see for ourselves that it is true both in our own experience and in the world around us. When it is time to embody the principle, we practice this new discipline until it becomes a passion. With the boundless energy of passion we practice this principle in all our affairs.

Reflection

Reflect on this process playing out in your own recovery. How have you gone from learning a discipline to living it?

153.

The four efforts are how we turn a passion for a principle into a skill that we can bring into each step we take. Our passion for recovery manifests in an appreciation for each principle, each practice that is supporting us as we take our first steps into a new life. Our recovery has made us a student of life principles. This experience has inspired us to experiment with them, practice them, live them. We bring our newfound principles to work with us and into our friendships; we even bring them home for the holidays.

The Buddha had nothing but admiration for this moment in a person's life. He called it entering the stream. He taught those who had entered the stream to watch the mind to see which mind states helped to achieve goals and which did not. He taught us to be sensitive, to see how we can be the change we want to see in the world by how we are taking this step. He taught us to see how we decide to take a step with our minds before the body actually moves. He taught us to nourish the mind. The Buddha believed the mind is like the body, that the mind is what we feed it. He taught us to watch what we feed the mind. This ultimately is what the four efforts amount to: a way to feed the mind properly.

Reflection

What are you feeding your mind these days?

Practicing Principles

In the next section, we will consider the ethical precepts that each of our three traditions sees as being required to succeed. Each tradition will offer us instruction on the intention with which we should take each step.

The first text used in 12-step programs came out in 1939. It bore the title *Alcoholics Anonymous* and became known as the *Big Book*. A second text, *Twelve Steps and Twelve Traditions*, which became known as the "12 and 12," was published in 1952 to help the growing global community of recovering people practicing the 12 steps laid out in the first text. In the "12 and 12," we are encouraged to "look squarely" at ourselves. We are told that "without a persistent and willing effort to do this, there can be little sobriety or contentment for us."

Once the recovering person has put down her substance or behavior, she is instructed to begin a mindfulness process to discover how she has been the author of suffering in her life. This process begins with a "fearless and thorough" inventory of her ethical lapses. This process is not as draconian as it sounds. Most newly sober people feel terrible about themselves in a way that is not sustainable. There needs to be a process early in recovery for putting an end to the supersized remorse of active addiction. This inventory allows the newly sober person to receive the wise, kind, nonjudgmental attention of someone who can give her a functional way to relate to her past. In addition to this fairly urgent need in early sobriety, the addict working her way through the inventory process begins to unravel cause and effect in her life. She gains insight in much the same way a meditator would as she observes the flow from mind state to behavior to consequence.

Reflection

Spoiler alert: all three traditions encourage you to look squarely at your behavior in an effort to unravel cause and effect in your life. All three offer specific instructions and practices to get this done. Each tradition offers us a bowl, and we must decide what to put into it. What bowls are you using these days? What are you putting into them?

155.

Having established that the root cause of our troubles are the habits of the mind, 12-step programs offer a mindfulness practice to observe these habits in action. This is a two-part process that begins with a written inventory of our behavior throughout the years, followed by a ritual in which the inventory is read to a trusted elder. The power of this process equals that of any mindfulness practice I have ever undertaken.

This process reflects the fourth and fifth steps of a 12-step program and follows the third step, in which the recovering person places her faith in the God of their understanding. Whether or not the word *God* is useful to you, it is important to understand what this step represents. When the Buddha sat, he systematically opened his heart before systematically opening his mind. The necessity of preparing the heart before examining the habits of the mind feels like an absolute we see across all disciplines. This absolute is reflected in the relationship between the third step and the fourth step. The recovering person prepares her heart before watching the mind.

Reflection

If we skip the heart, our efforts with our mind or our behavior will come to nothing. Can you be patient?

156.

The Buddha sat in an effort to understand himself. He noticed that when his heart opened, his mind became steady. He noticed that when his heart opened, his mind opened. The heart opens the door to understanding. The 12 steps begin with an in-depth study of the nature of the disease of addiction. Steps one and two identify the problem and suggest a solution in the same way the first three Noble Truths of Buddhism approach the phenomenon of human suffering. Step three prepares the heart for the difficult work ahead.

While yoga practices and Buddhism prepare the heart through meditation, 12-step programs prepare the heart through prayer. This prayer is to be taken both formally with a mentor and throughout the day when we want to make a new beginning. The Buddha encourages his students to abandon attachment; the third-step prayer allows the recovering person to abandon going it alone. The wording is from an explicitly theistic, patriarchal society in the grip of a centuries-long delusion of white supremacy, so there might be word choices to disagree with, but try to see the comfort it offers, the vulnerability it allows, the need for support it validates. Try to see the person asking for help.

> God, I offer myself to Thee to build with me as thou wilt. Relieve me of the bondage of self, that I may better do Thy will. Take away my difficulties, that victory over them may bear witness to those I would help of Thy Power, Thy Love, and Thy Way of life. May I do Thy will always!

Reflection

This prayer has provided me with a way to ask for help from life itself. How is your relationship to life these days? Do you feel you could ask it for help as you do the hard work of recovery? What would it mean to your heart if you felt life was on your side?

157.

Buddhism, yoga, and 12-step traditions prepare the heart for the difficult work of changing our minds. The emphasis in the 12-step tradition is on letting the individual know that she is not alone. The other two traditions prepare the heart by offering it the felt experience of kindness, compassion, joy, and equanimity. As the heart becomes accustomed to these states, it can call upon them when things get difficult. Twelve-step programs work with a traumatized population, and the focus is on a different set of felt experiences. The third step provides addicts with the felt experience of safety, of being held, of support, of refuge. As the addict's heart becomes accustomed to these states, she can call upon them when things get difficult.

Reflection

Can you see how the experience of safety will lead to the desire for joy?

158.

When I got sober, it became apparent that I had used a low-tech sedative to get through life. My early experience of life, without the ability to get numb, had been extremely raw. Sober, all of this rawness came back. I had tried to make the unacceptable acceptable because I had had no choice. The extent of that painful reality came rushing back as I sat through my first couple of years of 12-step meetings. I had had to make things okay that simply weren't. It wasn't okay that I had been subjected to abandonment and abuse. It wasn't okay that my society was in a frenzy of racial hate directed at people who looked like me. It wasn't okay that this was all I had ever known. It wasn't okay that I had not been up to the challenge. It wasn't okay that I'd had the living examples of MLK and Muhammad Ali but found myself unable to do more than try to get by. It wasn't okay that I had never been someone I could respect, let alone admire. None of it was okay.

The cultivation of compassion was not going to happen. I was in way too much pain for something so engaged. The preparation my heart needed was going to have to be very basic. I was not yet ready to believe in myself, but I had to be able to believe in life. At first, taking the third step felt false. I had a cell-deep aversion to religion. God felt like a disturbingly fanciful concept. And truth be told, I was never a joiner. But saying the third-step prayer when I ran up against my brokenness gave me a way forward. Each time I said the prayer, I felt how I was redefining my world. The third-step prayer states that I am in a world held by a divine presence invested in my progress whose plan I can be a part of. The third step prepared my heart by addressing my heartbreak. The third step let my heart believe in life again.

Reflection

What wasn't okay in your life? What can you do about it now? You will need to pick up the pieces and move on. But before that happens, the heart has to want to do so. Do you have the heart for this? Who can help you with your heart?

159.

One of the ways I have come to see the world is through the lens of the chakras, the body's energy centers. Each of our body's seven energy centers has a corresponding point of view. For example, the first chakra holds what we learned from our family, the second what we learned from our peer group, the third what we learned from our profession. Each perspective comes with a priority that shows up in our thinking about a situation. The first chakra wants to protect, the second chakra wants to have, the third chakra wants to prove. If I am trying to protect, have, or prove something at the same time, my body becomes gripped with tension. When this tension is present, I stop, relax, and then breathe the stuck energy up into my heart. My heart does not protect, have, or prove, so the tension leaves. When my body settles in this way, my mind clears.

With practice, I have come to feel perspective in my body. The heart's perspective is completely fearless because it is self-less. Without a self to worry about, we are free to have calm, clear awareness. The energy that is used to protect the self is released to be used in the service of our mental, emotional, physical, and spiritual well-being. All of this takes place in the space of a breath or two. All of this is why we prepare the heart before we try to change our mind.

Reflection

Sit still. Relax enough to be able to feel where your body is holding tension. Bring gentle awareness to this tension. While holding this tension in gentle awareness, begin to breathe the tension toward the heart. Let the whole space around the heart receive the tension. Hold the energy in your heart. What is it like when you move something into the heart?

160.

The role of ethical precepts in a spiritual practice is twofold. They prevent us from using our energy counterproductively while providing us with a mindfulness practice that focuses our attention on everyday life with ever-increasing subtlety. To do this work, we must prepare the heart. We must be our own best friend. Twelve-step programs do not expect you to be your own best friend at first. Nor do they feel it is prudent to wait until that happens before you start working on your recovery. Instead, they offer the newly recovering person a sanctuary of spiritual friendship in which to heal. There is a 12-step saying, "Let us love you until you can learn to love yourself." The mindfulness practice in a 12-step program is done in the presence of those who will love you until you can learn to love yourself.

Twelve-step programs provide the recovering person with three forms of spiritual friendship: meetings, sponsorship, and the God of your understanding. Each of these forms of friendship offers a different sort of intimacy. The type of spiritual friendship someone chooses is left up to the individual. The point is that she will not have to face herself alone.

Reflection

Consider the practical nature of an ethical precept: it allows you to avoid wasting time while cultivating an increasingly subtle connection to life. Now consider doing this with a friend. Can you think of a better way to bring spiritual practice into your everyday life?

161.

The terms *wise view*, *wise intention*, and *spiritual friendship* were used by the Buddha to describe the practices that needed to be in place before wise action could be attempted. Several thousands of years later, 12-step programs are putting these same practices in place before a recovering person embarks on the inner journey that will sustain her in her new life. The fourth and fifth steps of a 12-step program constitute the moment when the recovering person shifts her attention from her drinking problem to her living problem. She begins to bring a steady, nonjudgmental attention into her life. She starts with a written inventory of how the habits of her mind create the toxic emotional cycle that was the backdrop of her addiction.

Bill Wilson came up with a specific method to uncover the role of greed, hatred, and delusion in one's life. Addicts begin with a list of resentments—the ways you have resented this or that, what you don't like, and what you are holding on to. Then, with the help of a trusted mentor, you look squarely at how what you are holding on to has affected your life. Bill Wilson offered addicts a string to pull on that would in time unravel the entire process of holding on to our suffering in hopes that this time it will be different.

Reflection

You can get a sense of the power of the process by writing down a short list of your resentments right in this moment. Consider this list for a while. Does anything jump out at you?

162.

In some ways, the 12-step approach to ethics is to not approach it at all. Rather, it asks addicts to look at the cost of unskillful behavior. As a recovering person moves from step 4 through step 10, she first lists the ways she has been unskillful, then shares this list with someone she trusts. The next two steps are dedicated to using awareness, intention, and prayer to abandon her worst mental habits. To support this work, the addict makes a list of people who were harmed by her unskillful behavior, then makes direct amends to them "except when to do so would injure them or others." In the tenth step, she takes what she has learned from this immersion into her own behavior and conducts a brief inventory at the end of each day to see if any of her patterns have been at work. A key phrase from this daily inventory is "when we were wrong, promptly admitted it."

All of this amounts to a profound mindfulness practice that allows an addict to gain clarity about how she is moving through the world and gives her a chance to regain her self-respect. A person who is learning to live this way is being taught how to look at herself with an open heart and an open mind, seeking only to know what is true. Abraham Lincoln captured the spirit of these steps in the simple turn of phrase "with malice toward none, with charity for all."

Reflection

As we begin to look inside ourselves for answers, we find that we have "resigned from the debating committee." The dramas that used to distract us no longer have the same attraction. Inner peace becomes preferable to outer conflict. Are you starting to see evidence in this shift in your recovery?

163.

Getting sober meant that I had left my tribe. I was an outcast. My people were still drinking, and more important, they were still making excuses for their drinking. It was not only the effects of alcohol that I had left behind, but the thinking that made drinking necessary. It turns out my tribe was very attached to this kind of thinking, more so than they were to me. A stranger in a strange land, I gravitated to people who were going through what I was going through. In time, the stories of people who lived through a similar sort of transformation attracted me as well.

I noticed some common threads across time and culture:

1. When people find peace or God, the words are different but it amounts to the same thing.

2. People who find peace do not find it by getting the right things or having the right experiences. Peace comes to us in the form of a change in perspective. We see things in a way that we have not seen them before. This new seeing allows us to feel our heart's intention.

3. Everyone, everywhere, throughout all time, has described the heart's intention in the same terms. The heart is a sun that warms us through kindness, compassion, joy, and equanimity.

4. Life becomes a dance to the music of the heart.

Reflection

Is this true for you yet? Is recovery a dance to the music of your heart?

164.

People find peace. Some of us find it in the space of a breath, while others come to it slowly over time. I have been a bit of a hybrid. A sudden awakening through prayer got me sober. This sudden awakening has left me with what most people would describe as faith. It is not faith to me because I have had direct experience. Something lifted my addiction; during this interaction, I got a glimpse of its consciousness. It knows us completely. It loves us completely. It has only one job for us: to love each other the way it loves us. The problem for me was that its love is so mature, so compassionate, so unconditional. I felt the completeness of this form of love, I felt the injunction to give it a try 27 years ago. In my low moments, I have felt as if my efforts at loving this way resemble those of a four-year-old trying to build an airplane from instructions that he glimpsed on a billboard from a car window.

I could not build this love based on what I had glimpsed; I had to find people who were trying to build the same love. I had to find teachers. I had to find students. I had to teach what I was learning. I had to write books. For those of us trying to build love, communities teaching that the first step is to do no harm are particularly helpful. Love thrives in the absence of its opposite. Bill Wilson created this kind of community. The community that offered me my first yoga class was another.

Reflection

Write down a list of the qualities of the love you are building. Who is helping you with this?

165.

I began the practice of yoga the way many people do in the United States, in a group movement class. Because our tendency is to see what we expect to see, I found nothing particularly different about this movement class. There was a teacher and we did stuff. So what? Were it not for the fact that a yoga pose done even half right delivers profound energy healing, I would not have known anything at all about yoga after my first class. I had trained my body very hard for many years by the time I stepped onto my first yoga mat. An hour or two of group exercise was nothing new. What was new was what happened when I stepped off the mat.

In the past, after a workout, I carried tension in my body. The more intense the workout, the more tension I carried out of the gym. Some of my best workouts left me unable to drive. I would have to sit in my car for a while as the lactic acid that had built up in my arms slowly metabolized. After my first yoga class, the tension was not there. There was something else absent. Walking down the hall to breakfast, I could feel that the tension my body had held before class was gone as well. This was beyond new. This was rebirth.

Reflection

Imagine letting go of the past in your body. Yoga poses do that for you. Yogic breathing does it too. Why not give it a try?

166.

For a while, the fact that yoga made me feel better was more than enough incentive to practice daily. I also liked the ambience. Yoga was done in nice-smelling places with a spiritual vibe that did not feel religious. The atmosphere of a sacred space combined with the extremely cathartic poses was all I needed to feel that I had found a second spiritual community. I started spending my vacation time at a yoga center in western Massachusetts. Before long, it was all I wanted to do.

I attended a 30-day yoga teacher training as an excuse for spending part of the summer at my favorite place. The curriculum included talks on the Yoga Sutras. I have to say, they felt completely irrelevant to the process of doing yummy poses in a sacred space. Who needs a book when you are living it? The ethical precepts that were mentioned landed, however, because there were five of them. This offered me a structure that made sense. I had done the 12 steps, so why not try the five yamas? It felt pretty cool and yogaish to be committing to working on the yamas with the same dedicated mind-set that I had brought to the steps. The only problem was that there was no way to prepare my heart. Without a community, without a trusted mentor, without a higher power, it was just me trying to do something I did not really understand. The first thing I learned as I tried to practice the ethical precepts of yoga was that I would have to find the supports in yoga that I had in my 12-step program or I would never be able to do more than rock the physical poses while enjoying a sacred vibe. What had made the difference in my 12-step program had been the people; what had worked had been the relationships.

Reflection

If you are enjoying the poses, please do so for as long as you like. You have definitely earned a nice, long yoga honeymoon. If you are ready to go a little deeper, start looking at the relationships you are building within your yoga community. Are the others there to help you find the truth or just to have fun?

167.

A 12-step community benefits from the fact that the only people who are there need to be there desperately. This lends a sense of urgency to the process that translates into the pragmatic competence that is the hallmark of 12-step recovery. My meditation community benefits from the fact that its retreats are profoundly arduous for a newcomer. No one is going to meditate that long, that often, for days on end unless she is completely invested in the process. The arduous nature of the retreat tends to attract solid well-educated teachers. The excellence of the instruction combined with the investment of the students creates an indescribably impactful process.

The yoga community took off when the practice appealed to the group fitness crowd. This was not a small demographic. When they showed up, yoga went from a million people practicing several times a week to 25 million in 10 years. It's been a great thing for everyone involved. But the group fitness crowd is not in the market for change. They want the life they have right now, with maybe 10 pounds less, or maybe a little more free time. Some of my students want their husband to try yoga, and some of them want to leave their corporate job. But they definitely do not possess the sense of urgency that one sees at a 12-step meeting or the sense of purpose that someone needs in order to sit in meditation for many hours, day after day. The greatest obstacle the yoga community faces is the fact that it is a group of people who are doing all right. They are raising good kids, sending them to good schools, and working hard on their relationships. These are good people reaping the benefits of being good people. How do you get successful people to recognize the existence of suffering in their lives, let alone the need to undertake ethical training? I have found it helps to tell them the truth while teaching them to feel.

Reflection

Education is truth you can feel. Meetings make you feel. Yoga poses make you feel. Sitting still makes you feel. All you need to add to those situations is the truth. Where do you go to feel the truth?

168.

I learned my trade teaching yoga to large groups of people who were within walking distance of Harvard University. It was an extremely exposed sort of learning environment for a teacher. My classes would be full of Harvard grad students, fresh from lectures given by the best professors on the planet. As if that weren't bad enough, M.I.T. was two miles away, and Tufts was also within walking distance. Every time I stepped into my classroom, I was in the presence of serious intellectual horsepower. In the face of this much mental acuity, I had no choice but to stick to the truth. I am not sure that I could or would have taught any other way, but in this situation, it was clearly all I had to offer. Harvard Medical School professors did not need my take on human anatomy.

What I found with yoga students is that they respond to two things:

1. A challenge. It does not matter whether it is physical or spiritual. Yoga students get a certain light in their eyes if you respect them enough to challenge them.

2. Honor. I learned that it was not my role to preach. It was my role to remind students of their commitment to live honorably. Underneath the regular baggage of greed, hatred, and delusion that yoga students struggle with, you will find a bone-deep desire to live honorably. Yoga people get a certain light in their eyes when you challenge them to live honorably.

Reflection

Have you felt the excitement of finding yourself a part of a group of people who are accepting the challenge to live honorably? Is there anything better?

169.

With addicts, you start with the truth that their way isn't working at all. You are not telling them how to parent their children or giving them medical advice; you are just stating a plain fact they already know: *It only gets worse.* This is a hard truth that you can build on. With yoga students, you have to start with the truth that they have not yet learned how to let go. You are just stating a plain fact that they already know: *We cling to points of view that make us suffer.* This is a hard truth we can build on.

The physical process of a yoga class allows the student's struggle with attachment to be revealed. While sweating through a series of poses, a student's inner life is often a jumble of reactions. The "self's" struggle for control is laid bare in a situation that offers little in the way of control. Then, in a calm moment, I offer the students a chance to be still by letting stillness happen. They find that they can. They find that this is why they came. Then we sweat a little longer. In time, they return to one attachment or another, one preference or another, a self story, a reason to suffer. Then we are still, we let go again, we allow stillness to happen. Each time they let go, they feel their suffering cease. Each time they feel what ends their suffering, they are reminded of what causes their suffering.

Reflection

Stand or sit still. Then imagine you are a glass of water with sand stirred up in it. Now allow your sand to settle. Allow your water to become clear. Feel into your clarity. Do this throughout your day whenever your sand gets stirred up.

170.

Teaching yoga students offers some challenges that you will not see in my other two communities, but it also offers advantages that you will not see anywhere else. In yoga classes:

1. People stop to feel their breathing.

2. People move with calm care.

3. People feel the truth.

In yoga classes, people learn to feel the truth. The trick is to express the truth in a way they can feel. This was my learning process as a teacher: walking into a room day after day, finding ways to teach the truth in a way my students could feel. One of my favorite ways to teach the truth is to have people rest on the floor. As they settle, I tell them to "look directly at the relationship between letting go and receiving support, between letting go and being held by life."

Reflection

Rest comfortably on the floor, a couch, or your bed and feel the relationship between letting go and receiving support, between letting go and being held.

171.

For a while it is enough to feel into the present moment. Having spent as long as we can remember living in the dream world of our thinking, a breath or two in connection with the present moment feels miraculous. As the shift from attachment to connection becomes increasingly familiar to us, we start to notice that the two states have two value systems. In attachment, we are lacking; in connection, we are full. Each time we return to the experience of connection, we return to a worldview that is at peace. Each time we return to the experience of attachment, we return to a worldview that is in conflict. It is not subtle. One experience feels sacred. The other feels tormented.

At this point, we begin to take an active interest in the cultivation of the sacred. How can we spend more time in the sacred and less time in torment? What leads us to one? What leads us to the other?

Reflection

Make a list of moments that have felt sacred to you. Notice how often you were in nature. Notice how often you were connected to the world around you through the senses. What were the circumstances most closely associated with the sacred?

172.

Yogis sat in an effort to understand themselves. They noticed that when they connected to the present moment, their hearts opened. Staying with this experience, they noticed that when their hearts opened, their minds became still. Resting in connection, they spontaneously experienced kindness, compassion, joy, and equanimity. Drifting back into attachment, they spontaneously experienced greed, hatred, and delusion. Sitting in an effort to understand themselves, the Yogis observed the relationships between love and connection, fear and attachment.

Wanting the best for themselves, they learned to practice love. Wanting the best for themselves, they learned to abstain from the choices of fear. These choices became known as the yamas. Abstaining from them became the first practice of yoga.

Reflection

Love connects us; fear torments us. Can you place your trust in love? Can you turn your back on fear?

173.

A 12-step program teaches a recovering person the connection between attachment and relapse. Losing oneself in greed, hatred, and delusion is, as described in the A.A. Big Book, the "dubious luxury of normal men." For addicts, these states are a poison. Yogis observed the connection between attachment and suffering. They saw that there are habits of the mind that lead us down the path to suffering. They also saw that by abstaining from these mental habits, we free up energy that can be used to develop the habit of connection.

Like the ancient Yogi, the present-day 12-step participant responds to these insights by going on what Bill Wilson called a "fact-finding mission." Instead of simply trying to abstain from the habits of the mind that they have practiced all their lives, it makes more sense to get a feel for what has been going on. What helps? What hurts? For the 12-step person, this process is called the steps. For the Yogi, it is called meditation.

Reflection

The idea is that we put down our addiction so that we can pick up living. This process starts with a fact-finding mission. What helps? What hurts? Some people use the steps; others use meditation. What do you use?

174.

Because addicts tend to begin spiritual practice in response to a negative dynamic, we start our "fact-finding mission" in search of what causes suffering. Meetings work perfectly in this respect. There really is nothing like hearing another addict talk about her habit to get us in touch with what it was like to be at the mercy of an addiction. Meditation is a little subtler; at first the only cause of suffering seems to be meditation itself. Our back hurts, our knee hurts, time drags. After a while, our bodies are still troubled but our minds are the real problem. Sitting in meditation is a humiliating process in which we helplessly observe our mind running amok. What exactly is the point of this?

If we are willing to wade through the early days, we begin to see patterns. We notice that our mind is extremely repetitive, mulling over the same sorrows, the same infatuations, day after day. Eventually we start easing up. Maybe tolerating a childish, repetitive mind is as good as it gets? If we make it this far, we begin to have moments of true peace. The interruptions are not as unpleasant because we have accepted that "the mind moving is like this." We are patient when the mind moves because we have learned that it rests as well. Perhaps our first real meditative skill is the patience we need when the mind moves. We start to see that if we do not react to the moving mind, we will be more available for the moment when the mind stops. We have made a breakthrough. We have identified a positive mental state. We already knew that negative mental states made things worse; now we are seeing how certain other states make things better.

Reflection

The first thing meditation teaches us is patience. We learn that patience is an embodied choice. We become better at what we are doing or learning if we can be patient. Can you imagine how important it is for addicts to become good at patience? When would this be helpful?

175.

Time spent in meditation reveals two roads. One leads to suffering while the other leads to well-being. These roads do not exist in the physical world. They are roads that only the mind takes. On one road, the mind moves to create a self, then creates a world relative to the self it has created. On the other road, the mind rests in the experience of things as they are. On the first road, the relative world is further divided into pleasant and unpleasant, where the pleasant is wanted and the unpleasant is not. Meanwhile, on the second road, as the mind rests in the experience of things as they are, the heart opens. Life is difficult on the first road. In a world of things wanted or not wanted, there is no rest for the mind. With the mind in endless craving, the heart becomes increasingly irrelevant. This is the tragedy of ordinary consciousness. On the second road, the healing of the heart becomes the purpose of the resting mind. This is the miracle of meditation.

Reflection

If you know better, you do better. Knowing which road you are on is all that is necessary. When do you find yourself on the second road?

176.

In meetings, we observe the relationship between behavior and consequence. In meditation, we observe the relationship between mental states and behavior. Mental states lead to behavior, behavior leads to consequences, consequences are experienced as well-being or suffering. Wise action works in both directions. We practice wise action when we abstain from behaviors that lead to suffering. We practice wise action when we commit to behaviors that lead to well-being. These commitments have four types of effort:

1. Abstaining from negative behavior
2. Getting back on track when we have fallen into negative behavior
3. Cultivating positive behavior
4. Sustaining healthy habits once they have been established

We also practice wise action when we are willing to reflect on the state of mind we were in before we took an action that led to suffering. The same is true when we reflect on the state of mind we were in when we took an action that led to well-being. This reflection leads to four types of effort:

1. Steering clear of negative mind states
2. Getting unstuck when we get stuck in negative mind states
3. Cultivating positive mind states
4. Maintaining positive mind states once they are established

Reflection

Wise action works in both directions. Choose one negative behavior to drop and one positive behavior you wish to add at the same time. As you work on this, notice which mind states help and which ones do not.

177.

Wise action works in both directions. The first time I was taught this explicitly was when I was told "Don't drink" *and* "Go to meetings." I complied on both counts out of desperation. I was not thinking of the larger implications in terms of how spiritual practice works; I was just trying to avoid an alcoholic death. Not drinking felt like half of the equation. Without the support of meetings, not drinking did not seem remotely possible. Going to meetings felt like the other half of the equation. Without the extreme challenge of life without alcohol, meetings would not have possessed the same relevance. Taken together, the two actions amounted to an extremely wise choice for someone dying of an addiction.

Once I got to a meeting, I would spend some time listening and some time talking. After meetings, I'd spend some time with my sponsor and some time with new folks I was sponsoring. Once I got home, I would spend some time in prayer and some time in meditation. The next day I would go to my job, where the waiters were taught to work together. We were told to ask for help and to give help. Wise action works in both directions.

Reflection

There is a push among those getting sober to limit wise action to simply not drinking. "Just don't drink" is a sort of battle cry for those who do not wish to do more, as if all the pieces of a good life will arrange themselves for us if we just don't drink. Wise action encompasses both what we are abandoning and what we are cultivating. A person in recovery is stepping out of a life of addiction into a life of connection.

178.

As a yoga student, I was taught wise action in a systematic fashion. It began with how I held my body in a pose. Then I was taught how to breathe in a way that settled the mind. I was taught the wisdom of an undistracted mind, a directed mind, a settled mind, a mind that has let go. Each of these teachings was a form of action in which I was both steady and relaxed. The body was steady and relaxed. The breath was steady and relaxed. The attention was steady and relaxed. The will was steady and relaxed. The heart was steady and relaxed. Wise action worked in both directions.

As I tried to learn this, I would lean toward too much steady and not enough relaxed. I trusted working hard, but I did not trust letting go. Letting go did not offer me the ability to be in control, to be safe, or to be sure. I had combined not drinking with meetings because I was desperate. On a yoga mat or a meditation cushion, I had to learn to work in both directions for another reason. I had to want more for myself than trying to fly with just one wing. This required self-respect. It required self-compassion. It was a process that took many years, but I got there because people kept reminding me that I was worth it until I remembered.

Reflection

Where in your life are you trying to fly with just one wing?

179.

My meditation teachers taught me that there were two limbs of practice. They said that the cultivation of wisdom and compassion taken together were like the two wings of a bird creating the possibility of flight. One would not work without the other. For a number of years, I was not ready to hear this. I wanted wisdom. I wanted to be smarter than the disease of addiction. I sat in meditation in an effort to understand myself but did not see how self-compassion offered more than a set of excuses. I thought I was done with excuses. Sitting day after day in an effort to understand myself, I became aware of my patterns. I saw them, I judged them, and I judged myself for having them. I felt I was done with excuses, but I could not see a way forward that did not entail being someone else. One year, I was taught self-forgiveness. I was taught to see the behavior and the person as two different things. In this fashion, I was able to sit with a life of mistakes. I was able to sit with a life of imperfections. I was able to sit with a life of learning. I saw that I am the way forward. I knew what it meant to be done with excuses. Wise action works in both directions.

Reflection

Imagine that being kind to yourself was the beginning of wisdom. What would that mean?

Chapter Five

Service

Bill Wilson sat with Dr. Bob Smith in an effort to understand himself. Together they discovered that by helping another addict, an individual could overcome what had been a fatal illness. This insight became the basis of the 12-step program they founded. Fifteen years later, a very sick Dr. Smith gave his last talk at a 12-step convention. He felt that the purpose of his words was to remind his listeners of what they already knew, that the 12 steps came down to love and service. He said, "We understand what love is, and we understand what service is." Let's keep this in mind as we offer the next person the same sort of aid that we received in our own hour of need.

In this section we look at the power of helping others.

180.

We begin with one life. We save one life when we stop using. For some of us, that will be all. I worked for a while with addicts who had stopped using as they were going through the process of dying from AIDS. These people were offering themselves love and freedom at the end of their lives. Saving a life. It was enough.

Others of us stumble through the first few months of not using only to realize that there are many miles to go before we sleep. What are we to do with this future we never thought we would have?

The year after I got sober, I watched spring bring color back into the world with eyes that could see. Sitting with a friend in the lingering light of a late-spring evening, I experienced speechless awe. I was in awe of the freedom. I was in awe of the good fortune. Sitting in the warmth of that exquisite light, I saw how many spring evenings lay before me. How do I use this gift? How do I spend this time in a way that expresses my gratitude? How do I tell the world what it means to me to have the spring back?

Reflection

What is your favorite season? What does it mean to have it back?

181.

I tried to help out. I took volunteer positions at meetings. I volunteered at the local Audubon Society. When I went to work, I made an honest effort at making the lives of those around me easier. At meetings, I tried to share in a way that was constructive. In my relationships, I made every effort to apply what I was learning in meetings. These were things people told me to do. They were good things. My heart was full, and it demanded action, any action that was loving.

Within just a few years, I began seeing people who offered me something much bigger. They were dedicating their professional lives to expressing the spirit of our community. My recovering community had taught me that full human potential is reached when we affirm each other. We cannot do it alone, but if we do it together, anything is possible. I saw that people could bring this spirit into the world. Their title could be teacher, or police officer, or governor, but the impact of their efforts was to give the world a sense of what we were learning in meetings about love and service. This spoke to me. I felt a bone-deep desire to use my work life to share what I had learned about people helping people.

Reflection

What speaks to you?

182.

There was a period of calibration. My second 12-step mentor was in medical school. He encouraged me to follow in his footsteps. I went back to school, became an emergency medical technician, then began taking premed courses. I enjoyed the course work, but my experience of working full-time on an ambulance was not exactly what I was looking for. I liked the challenge. I liked caring for people. I liked working with a partner. But there was something missing.

I was working in Boston, so the variety of calls I got was endless. One moment I would be transporting someone to dialysis, the next I would be assisting paramedics as they tended to someone in the middle of a heart attack. When addicts need to get help for their addiction, they often begin their journey at an ER. Stabilized from whatever medical emergency brought them in, the lucky ones get sent to a rehab or detox facility. I often found myself bringing people from an ER to an addiction-treatment facility. These calls seemed to happen in the dead of night. Someone in shock would be brought from the bustle of an urban ER to the relative quiet of an inpatient treatment facility. The check-in process would be brief; then they would go to their room. In the odd deep darkness that exists several hours after midnight, I would talk to the counselors about their work with addicts.

Reflection

We have to be willing to act on behalf of our hearts that are longing to serve long before we know how it is going to work out. What is your heart's longing? Are you waiting to know how it will work out?

183.

During the time I was going to school to become an emergency medical technician, I bought a book on meditation. It was the early 1990s, and this type of book was very much in fashion. There were several bookstores within walking distance of one of my favorite meetings. One of the bookstores I liked most was rectangular, a traditional affair with windows that brought in New England's seasons. Another encompassed several floors perched on a bend of a busy street. I was in this second one when I ran across a book called *Zen Mind, Beginner's Mind*. It was short with a cool Zen-ish cover.

The author wrote brief essays that were a perfect length for someone to read before sitting to meditate. I would read something that I did not really understand, then count breaths for twenty minutes. The process was entirely satisfactory. I was working hard to increase my love and service game. I wanted to bring what I was learning into the world. I was young and active, but somehow sitting quietly, counting breaths, made a huge difference. Without needing to think much about it, I stayed with it.

Reflection

Our destiny often shows up when we aren't looking for it. Without our really asking it to, it sticks around. Is anything sticking around for you these days?

184.

There are turning points. My first year of premed courses went well. (Being a sober student felt as good as it sounds.) As the summer approached, I had to make a decision. I could take my final requirements in an expensive flurry of summer courses. This would put me in position to apply to medical school in the fall. Or, for less money than I would spend on summer school, I could take a three-semester course that would qualify me to work as an addictions counselor.

My late-night talks with addictions counselors were making me reconsider my commitment to medical school, but so was something else. Going to meetings was teaching me to want the best for myself. I was learning to trust enough to try, to dare, to take a leap of faith. I was learning faith. Sitting in meditation was teaching me to sit in truth. Faith and truth were becoming part of how I was living. I was seeing with faith and truth mixed in. I was listening with faith and truth mixed in. I was learning to choose with faith and truth mixed in. I talked it over with a dear friend. I met with my mentor. I told him about my faith in truth. That fall, I went to school to become an addictions counselor.

Reflection

What is it like to be living with faith and truth mixed in?

185.

There are signs. I was staying sober through a combination of meetings, meditation, ethical precepts, and service. It was a good period in my life. The disciplines I had embraced were adding up to an optimistic, engaged sort of sobriety that I was enjoying immensely. Around this time, my future wife came into my life. She was someone whose approach to life I respected completely. She went away for a weekend to spend some time at a place I did not really understand. Apparently people went there to enjoy themselves in a peaceful, contemplative sort of way. When she came back, she brought a fall-colored leaf the size of a dinner plate.

Going to meetings had made me sensitive to the concept of possibility. Active addicts lose heart. Part of this is losing touch with the possibilities all around them. Going to meetings had reawakened my sense of adventure. Sitting in meditation had profoundly affected the acuity with which I could experience something. Looking at that leaf, I felt a sense of possibility that included how meditation had touched my heart. The stillness of meditation also allowed me to sense the aura of peace that surrounded this leaf. I wanted to see the forest this leaf had called home. I asked my new friend to tell me where she had found such a leaf. Mariam replied that it came from the Kripalu yoga center.

Reflection

They say that when the student is ready, the teacher will appear. Our job is to get ready. This is what a program of recovery really is. It is how we get ready for the adventure of a lifetime. How are you getting ready?

186.

There is synchronicity. The work I was doing with ethical precepts supported my path of service. There is a consistency to our behavior when it is in alignment with life's basic laws. Non-harming, honesty, kindness, and compassion never go out of style. By combining the practice of ethical precepts with a commitment to serve others, I found myself in the right place at the right time permanently. Ethical precepts offer us the chance to look honestly at the choices we are making. When looked at honestly, there is no better choice than spending our days in work that expresses our compassion for human suffering. There is no greater joy than to know, really know, that our efforts have lessened someone's load, that someone remembers our kindness.

I was not confused about this as I began working in the addictions treatment field. My 12-step community had taught me in no uncertain terms that we get what we give. As the days went by, however, it turned out I had overlooked something. The underlying premise of my plan was that if I took care of others, life would take care of me. Life did in fact do its part. My heart kept beating. Opportunities mounted. Grace occurred regularly, but it was not life's job to do what I needed to do for myself. It was my job to make sure I got enough sleep, that I nourished myself physically, emotionally, and spiritually. One of the first things I learned on my path of service was that I could not give what I did not have. If I was not learning to be happy, I could not teach others to choose happiness. At this exact moment in my life, Mariam brought home a leaf from the leading yoga center in the United States.

Reflection

Can you see how ethical commitments and the commitment to serve others support each other? Do you see that you can't give what you do not have?

187.

For a while, it was enough to spend my days helping young people find their way out of addiction. I worked the second shift. As night fell, the children I worked with did homework, ate dinner, then participated in an evening activity. There were groups to lead; twice a week I took the young addicts I cared for to 12-step meetings. I also had counseling responsibilities. It was a full day that ended at midnight. I would ride my bike home through the darkened streets of Cambridge. The next day would be more of the same.

By this time I already had several practices in place to get me ready for work. I loved reading books on living skillfully, so I was always in the middle of one. The comfort these books gave me cannot be put into words. I would read for a while, then sit in meditation. At noon I would attend a 12-step meeting within walking distance of my house. As the time to leave for work approached, my body would become tense. This physical tension would be accompanied by a growing dread. I did not have mental anguish, nor was I dreading something in particular. I just had the habit of getting tense and feeling dread. I found that spending time on my mat helped. A lot. After a while, I did not mind my habit of dreading because I knew what to do. The yoga poses not only released the tension and dread but replaced them with an energetic optimism. At some point, I stopped feeling dread altogether. Long before that, I had noticed the tension of dread in the children I worked with, as well as in the people at my meetings. I saw how everyone, everywhere carried the tension of fear in their bodies because it was all they had ever known.

Reflection

Yoga poses are a response to the human habit of carrying tension in our bodies. Addiction is another. What is your response?

188.

My practice became a combination of not drinking, going to meetings, working with ethical precepts, serving others, reading spiritual teachings, cultivating spiritual friendships, and practicing meditation and yoga. I should also mention that spending time in nature, exercising or just appreciating it, has been a constant throughout my recovery. (I am writing this book in a redwood forest that overlooks the Pacific Ocean.) It has not been hard to manage this array of activities because it is all I have wanted to do. It is the why and what of my sobriety. If I stopped teaching yoga tomorrow, my life would not change in any way except that I would have to find another way to share what I share in yoga classes. My disciplines are my passions. My passions are my life.

I experience service as the moment when I see how others can benefit from what I have learned. It is a unique form of intelligence to recognize how we can help someone; I do not take it for granted. What I like better, however, is the challenge of finding a way to teach what I love, to transform my learning process into a teaching process that becomes a new learning process. For me, this is being in life to the fullest extent.

Reflection

Has a discipline of recovery become a passion for you?

189.

My time as an addictions counselor was spent in the belief that I would never be doing anything else. I had looked very deeply into what I wanted to do for a living. Addictions treatment was my first choice. I went to school for it, paid my dues, did my part. My first couple of years managed to be both extremely low paying and tremendously difficult. There was a trip to Mount Washington during which one of my students took the wrong path and got into a van with strangers. The state police called to tell us the nice people in the van had dropped the student off at a hostel 10 miles away. Then there was the evening I found myself on the roof of our facility looking down upon an army of fire trucks while I talked to a student about why he wanted to come off the ledge. There was a family that lost a child. My heart was broken many times, but I never lost sight of the sacred nature of people helping people. My sobriety allowed me to be held by the power of our common humanity while I made the first honest effort in my life.

Reflection

How are you allowing others to help you do your best?

190.

I was making an honest effort at learning how to help young addicts. It was paying off. I was getting better at it. After a few years, I was accepted into a prestigious graduate program. I became the president of the student government. The dean of students asked me if I would consider getting my doctorate. It all felt good. Yoga felt better. I loved the devotional feeling of it. Placing my hands on the mat in downward dog has always felt like remembering connection. *I am connected to the earth. I am connected to all beings. I am connected to God. I come back to this. I touch the earth.* I knew where my heart was, but I struggled with guilt. My work in the addictions field was raw, hard, messy, courageous. Yoga was safe, quiet, with the potential to be escapist. It also had the potential to change the world in a way that had never been seen before. The good was fighting hard with the best.

With each passing day, I found my heart leaping more toward yoga and less toward working in chinos with a plastic badge whose purpose was to say that I was not like my clients. I loved the earthy simplicity of yoga, the physical nature of it, the spiritual nature of it. I loved the fact that we were exploring emotions in stillness rather than with words. I loved the fact that we were working with trauma in our bodies rather than in our stories. I loved the fact that we were coming home, that we were remembering. But I was not ready to leave the world I had fought so hard to be a part of. I had started teaching a yoga class at my graduate school. Then I discovered that I could support myself during my clinical placements by teaching yoga. It was more than I could bear to take the journey, but I could take a step, and then another step.

Reflection

If you do not feel ready to take the journey, are you willing to take a step?

191.

We need each other. We need the spaces we create together. We need each other's stories to understand our own. We need each other's wisdom. We need each other's compassion. We need each other's imagination and our collective ability to envision a better way. I learned this in meetings. I had this same lesson reinforced in great detail by my experiences in the addictions treatment field. If our *default* is to drift into a state of craving that is so intense that we start seeing backward, our collective *potential* is to live into the idea of "on earth as it is in heaven."

As I began moving people through yoga classes, this sense of our default setting and our actual potential hovered about in my subconscious. What I had seen had given me great faith in human potential, but I did not possess an in-depth theory of how a yoga class fit into that potential. The same was true in the negative. I was aware of our tendency to fall into craving and delusion, but I could not tell you in any factual way how yoga offset this default. I just knew that yoga moved people in a way that felt very important. I would go to class and work with them. Encourage them. Affirm them. Move the process along. When a class was over, we all felt as if something important had happened. It became my calling to work with others to create this thing we all agreed was important but could not name.

Reflection

As far as I can tell, we all share the same default setting, which we fall back into when the right circumstances arise. Our actual potential feels a little more particular. You will flower in this way; someone else will flower in another way. This flowering happens when the right circumstances arise. Love is essential. What pushes you into your default? What pushes you into your potential?

192.

My 40s were hard until I learned the importance of having a hobby. The practice of having a hobby gives an adult the chance to keep learning new things with people who share a common interest. Research suggests that without embracing new disciplines by learning new skills, the mind starts to slide toward dementia in one's 50s. I believe a part of the phenomenon of the middle-aged passion for hobbies is biologically driven. We need to keep learning to keep living. My own experience is that hobbies allow me to find common ground with people I would not ordinarily feel I had anything in common with. The value of learning new skills while meeting new people who possess different worldviews is obvious.

This refreshing experience first came to me in the form of surfing. I grew up in the frozen north. My time in the ocean before surfing could be counted in hours, not days. My time in pools, however, could be counted in decades. The combination of being utterly ignorant of the ocean yet utterly at home in the water gave me all I needed for a wondrous multiyear learning adventure.

My next hobby was inspired by my son's success in wrestling. Dylan showed promise early on. The athletes were amazing young people, but what really interested me was how the coaches were developing human potential. Their job is very similar to mine, and studying how they approach it has become my new passion. Over the next few essays, I will use what I am learning from wrestling coaches to contextualize the experience of teaching yoga as one's path of service. For this essay, I will leave you with some highlights:

1. Good coaches teach people to focus on the effort, not the result.

2. Good coaches teach their athletes to "wrestle free," which means to wrestle with non-attached enjoyment. Teams that win have learned how to do this.

3. The best team in college wrestling practices gratitude and joy as a way of life.

Reflection

Imagine approaching the most challenging situations in your life with gratitude and joy.

193.

An elite college wrestling coach's job is entirely about results; it is about winning. The kids they work with have been exceptional at winning. The kids' families, their communities, and the tens of thousands who fill the arenas all want to see them continue winning. It is in this potentially toxic environment that the best coaches have taught young people to value principle, process, and effort over results. The consistency with which the best wrestlers talk about this shift in perspective is dramatic. When asked how they get up for matches, they say that they just remember to be grateful for the opportunity. When asked how they come back from an early-season loss, they say that a win or a loss does not have the power to define them as a person. When asked what they want from an important tournament, they will say that too much emphasis is placed on winning. They will say that their preparation, their visualization, and their intention are focused on giving a full effort every second of every period. They will say that their hearts' desire is to be who they know they can be and to wrestle free.

When I think of the effect I want yoga to have on the world, it would be to have everyone talk about their life in this way.

Reflection

One of the ways we come back from addiction is to remember that a win or a loss does not have the power to define us. What matters is a full effort. You know you've put in a full effort when your heart is at peace. How is your heart today?

194.

Wrestlers get into trouble in big matches when they get "tight," which means they start wrestling to protect a lead or to avoid losing. The Buddha would have called this getting caught in a contracted state. The best wrestling coaches do not teach their athletes to avoid getting tight; they teach their athletes to wrestle free. These coaches teach that winning a match is the mountain you are climbing; wrestling free is the intention with which you take each step. They teach their young people that to wrestle free in the most important matches of your life, you have to wrestle free in the least important moments in practice. You have to wrestle free in your schoolwork, your friendships, in the difficult moments and in the joyous ones. These coaches do not believe you will wrestle free unless you live free. To teach this, I have had to learn to live it.

Reflection

It is said that we are what we habitually do. The great coaches are teaching their athletes to wrestle free by living free. If you were your own coach, what would you be teaching?

195.

In my first year of teaching yoga, I was still in graduate school. I taught in very small settings, so the only pressure was the pressure I put on myself. There was no one to compare myself with, and no way to fail. I just showed up and performed an extremely humble service for people who were very nice about it. The following year I became the director of Boston's first big yoga studio, teaching classes that averaged 60 to 80 people. It was uproariously high-visibility, high-stakes yoga teaching. That year all of the major newspapers and magazines in Boston ran stories on us. Within the next couple of years, *People* magazine, *Yoga Journal*, and *Travel + Leisure* would follow suit.

My first lesson in this bonfire of the vanities was to find a way to not take myself too seriously. It was next to impossible. Every mistake I made, every foolish comment, every moment of incompetence in the midst of a very steep learning curve happened in front of what felt like my entire community. I thought working with kids was difficult. Working with my own fear of rejection was way harder. When I focused on the results, my inner life was an emotional roller coaster. These emotional ups and downs left me drained and my performance suffered, which led to more emotional turmoil. Eventually I learned to remember the sacred nature of what was happening in the classes. I would spend time before class visualizing how I wanted people to feel as they walked back onto the street after class. I allowed myself to feel the comfort yoga was providing them. By remembering the beauty of the process, I could focus on my part, my effort. It began with the effort to be courageous in class, to be honest, to be kind. Then it became the effort to be a good husband, a good father, a good friend. At some point being a good student became very important; at another point, being a good friend to myself did as well. At each turn I have been reminded that if I want to teach from a place of freedom, I have to live from one.

Reflection

Is there an area of your life where you know what it means to live free?

196.

A way to understand my learning process as a yoga teacher is to imagine my delusional self-concept as a statue standing between me and a class that I am teaching. Then imagine that I am complaining about how difficult it is to see the class. Your job in this scenario would be to help me see the class. Your first gambit might be to have me move, but when I do not stop complaining, you notice that although I have moved my body, my eyes have never left the statue. At that point you would gain the insight that it is not where I stand that matters. It's where I place my attention. Your next strategy might be to suggest that I would be more successful if I stopped looking at the statue. This seems reasonable, but instead of thanking you I tell you that I am looking at the whole class, which includes the statue. Your work begins in earnest when you realize that I do not know that the statue is not a person.

You embark on a series of questions to determine just how real I think this statue is. You ask why I think the statue is relevant to the experience of the students. It becomes clear that I am trapped in a delusional relationship with the statue. I resist every effort you make to convince me of this. You realize that how I see things makes sense to me. You observe that, in addition to harboring a delusional perspective on the statue, I cling tenaciously to my point of view. There is just no talking to me. So you stop. Instead of asking me to look away from the statue, you ask me to feel my feet on the floor. While I'm rooted in the sensations of my feet, you suggest that I feel the in breath and then the out breath. It seems to help. You continue in this vein, teaching me to bring my movements into harmony with the rhythm of my breath. During a quiet moment in this process, you notice that I have begun teaching the students to feel their feet.

Reflection

At 12-step meetings, you are told to develop sober feet. The idea is that if you bring the body, the mind will follow. You are also taught that if you move a muscle, you will change a feeling. Yoga teaches both practices. Zen teachers say that to take the right posture is to take the right frame of mind. You can trust your body to bring you into the moment, and the moment to bring you into freedom. Try it now. Sit still, breathe, and let go.

197.

So there has been the work I've had to do to get over myself in order to be of service. Putting what this has been like into words is difficult. An analogy that comes to mind is being asked to groom a giant, unruly meadow with a child's plastic scissors. It's not impossible, but really . . . ? Imagine all of the moments you would want to throw down your idiotic little scissors and go home. Imagine something so compelling that you never do, not once. In addition to the challenge of getting out of my own way, there is the fact that until I did, my ability to know what was happening around me was impaired. I was required to lead with a distorted sense of what was necessary. I had to make do.

Like someone who has lost the ability to see, you learn to listen, to feel, to smell, to taste so you can make sense of your world. Instead of sight, what someone loses when caught up in the false self is empathy. Lacking empathy, I had to reality-test. Lacking empathy, I would watch the students' lungs moving under their ribs to see how much effort they were putting forth. Lacking empathy, I became adept at reading body language, reading the type of sweat—was it beading or coming down in sheets? Lacking empathy, I watched how fast the legs went into the air an hour into class. Lacking empathy, I listened closely to the sound of the *Om* at the end of class. Empathy gives us information directly; lacking it I had to get my information indirectly. Gathering information indirectly takes time. Yoga teaching becomes art when you no longer need time.

To be who I was born to be, I had no choice but to find what was beyond making do.

Reflection

Addicts are excellent at making do, but we can move beyond it. How are you making do? How can you move beyond it?

198.

There was never a moment when I did not want to do better. The magnificent possibility of a yoga class was my opportunity, my chance to be an artist. I was not going to win an Oscar or an Olympic gold medal. I would not hit the beaches on my generation's D-day. I would not walk with MLK or die with those who walked up the stairs of a tower as it went up in flames. I will not be remembered, but what I was a part of will. Yoga will be what future generations know about me, what I believed in, what I hoped for, what I fought for. We are yoga's chance. Yoga will be what we make of it.

Reflection

Our survival, our recovery, our community, our love, our service will be what future generations will know about us. Recovery is our chance. And we are recovery's chance. You may not have chosen this path, but it has chosen you. What will you make of it?

199.

There has never been a moment when I have not been grateful to have something worth getting better for. Better at leading. Better at learning. Better at loving. This has been the light in my life, the light that gives me a purpose, a path, the possibility of honor. It would be enough to have this light.

But then someone comes along to help.

Reflection

Survival is enough of a purpose—to show up sober at a graduation, a wedding, a funeral. This is enough. The heart rests. Then a task is placed in our hands, something that only we can do. When we take it up, a light enters the world.

200.

There were a number of years when I just tried harder. I taught thousands of classes during this time. Years went by. I woke up, practiced yoga, taught yoga. The next day I would review what I had taught the night before, feeling it in my body as I practiced. That night, I would teach again. The next morning I would review what I taught. I was sober, and I was helping people with the pain in their lives.

I was driven by what happened when we broke through. We would show up as a group of separate individuals, but at some point the group would become a unified field of energy. For a while, we would be everything that has ever worked about being human. For an exquisite moment, I would not feel disappointed at being the person God had dragged from a death that I had been sprinting toward. For a while, I would not have to feel the disappointment in my parents' eyes. For a while, I could forget how I felt about myself. Then it would be over. I would say goodnight to people whose eyes were still lit by what had happened. There would be a few moments of contentment, a sense of awe at what I'd been a part of. But walking back out into the night, these feelings would begin to fade. The loneliness would start to come back. As I walked through city streets, I would look into restaurants feeling separate from the happy faces. I had succeeded in becoming sober. I had succeeded in becoming a teacher. But I had not succeeded in becoming comfortable in my own skin.

Reflection

As active addicts, we have had to make do without the ability to be comfortable in our own skin. This feeling continues into sobriety. Having dealt with it in active addiction, we continue to make do in sobriety. Are you willing to settle, or are you willing to do something about it?

201.

The problem was that I was attempting to assert control over my life from the outside in. I worked hard so that I could get a specific outcome. I often accomplished my goals. But none of my accomplishments changed how I felt about myself. I was so certain that if I achieved this or that, I would be able to make peace with myself. Then the day would come. I would have a brief high followed by loneliness, disappointment, and the sense that surely if I accomplished a little more, I would be okay. This would have been a difficult dynamic in any person's recovery. Living it while leading thousands of people in spiritual practice was unmanageable.

There is a consequence, which is the result of a behavior, which is the result of a mind state. There is only so much you can do while working at the first two levels. Eventually you have to work directly at the level of mind states. This is the "why" of seated meditation. By sitting still, we relinquish behavior. We relinquish control. In the complete absence of behavior and control, we can give our undivided attention to our mind states. It seems simple enough, but the suffering most humans endure on a daily basis makes asserting some control seem preferable. Who has time to sit down and do nothing, with so much suffering to deal with? This was my predicament. Then someone came along to help.

Reflection

Watch what happens when you do nothing, how the mind still moves. This movement is what gives rise to behavior, which gives rise to consequences. Watch the mind move.

202.

As an addict, I tend to struggle with the choice between making do and solving a problem. If you can make do, why go to the trouble of actually addressing the problem? So I made do for a long time, feeling better during class, then slowly slipping back into my broken relationship with myself. My sporadic attempts at getting better tended to be aimed at a little more control—over my food, my time, my money, my body. This wouldn't pan out, so I would go back to making do. This dynamic was not without consequence. It meant that I was limited in my ability to help people. You cannot give what you do not have. During the transcendent moments in class, I caught glimpses of what could be. I even felt my ability to channel perfect wisdom, the flawless orchestration of movement, breath, intention. But that was the extent of it, just a glimpse. Once the moment was over, I was back to being me.

After a painfully long time in this state of affairs, a friend from the West Coast called me. He was in town because he had been attending a meditation retreat outside Boston. I was glad to hear from him; he was a good friend. He said the retreat had been magical. I thought that sounded pretty good. Nothing I had done had really worked, so maybe I should try doing nothing.

Reflection

Try doing nothing. Spend time in silence—no reading, no music, no journaling. Only silence. Then try spending time in silence in nature.

203.

Meditation teachers tell us that there are two parts to our practice: sitting quietly and sweeping the garden. As I have reflected on this teaching, I have turned it into a circle. Spiritual practice (sitting quietly) opens our heart. Our heart demands a path of service (a garden to sweep) that is worthy of it. If we are sweeping a garden worthy of our heart, we will be inspired to sit quietly with all of the skill and heart we can summon. Our practice opens our heart, our heart demands a life worthy of it, our life demands practices that are worthy of it.

When my friend called to tell me about his meditation retreat, I was sweeping a garden worthy of my heart. His call let me know it was time to find a practice worthy of the classes I was leading and the life I was living. Just as my sobriety had led me to my yoga mat, my yoga mat led me to my meditation cushion.

Reflection

If your recovery has opened your heart, are you listening to it? If so, what garden would it have you sweep?

204.

Combining sobriety with a path of service gives us our best shot at staying teachable. A path of service without a spiritual practice can easily lead to burnout, complacency, or codependence. A spiritual practice without a path of service is like getting all dressed up with no place to go. But together they create a life second to none.

This was the good news as I walked home through the darkened streets of Boston and New York looking at the happy faces in the restaurants. I was sober, I was doing all that I knew how, and I was helping others. With these factors in place, there was a strong probability that I would not settle for making do. There was also a strong possibility that someone would come by to help. The suffering contained in those moments did not lead to despair. Instead it led to a willingness to try something new, take a risk, let go.

Reflection

With the right factors in place, our lives become a series of predictable miracles. But don't take my word for it. Stay sober, try a few disciplines, and see what happens. Reflect on your recovery so far. Have you had any miracles?

205.

I showed up at my first meditation retreat with the skills I had picked up over 15 years of sobriety, skills that had been refined in the crucible of addictions counseling. I had also spent the past 10 years practicing and teaching yoga. Knowing a lot can be a challenge when it comes to learning something new. The offset for knowing too much is to put what you know to the test by trying to help someone. Helping others keeps us humble. Facing life's endless diversity, life's endless challenges in the form of the people we are serving, reveals the limits of our knowledge on a daily basis.

A friend of mine who is literally a rocket scientist at NASA says that in her world, the more you know, the more you know you don't know. As her team plans to create a new space station to support trips to Mars, they struggle with the uncertainty about the amount of uncertainty they need to plan for. When I sat down for my first day on a meditation retreat, the fact that I had put what I had learned to the test of service meant that it was usable knowledge. It was practical wisdom I could use to learn more. I was pretty certain about the amount of my uncertainty. All I was going to have to change was the way I thought about everything.

Reflection

In the last chapter, we discussed honest effort. In this section, we are examining the role of service to others on a path of recovery. Service can help us put our disciplines to the test. Time spent in the service of others gives us a reality-based recovery. How do you test the beliefs that you are cultivating in recovery?

206.

Getting sober was the greatest challenge I have ever faced. I dug deep, but the alternative was an addict's death. The remainder of the hardest challenges I have ever met were sustained by the fact that they were expressions of my commitment to service.

Before I got sober, long before my first meditation retreat, I went to the U.S. Army Ranger School. The conditions Ranger students endure are as close to sustained combat operations as possible. During my time there, we were allowed no more than three hours of sleep and one meal per day. We were given 10 meals in bulk every 10 days but usually ate most of the allotment in the first 3 days. The seven days that followed were a challenge. The sleep came after we had finished all our duties. This meant the actual amount of sleep we were getting was around an hour a day. If we were in a leadership position, we got none. At one point, because I went through Ranger School as an officer, I spent seventeen days in a row in leadership positions.

I was in Ranger School for 81 days. During my first four weeks, I thought about how I was doing, when I would get out, and what I would do when I got home. The rest of my time there, I focused on the step I was taking, the set of my rucksack, the ease with which I could manage an incline or decline. I learned to take comfort in the support I could offer those around me. We came to truly value each other, to think and act as a team in everything. When I graduated, I was as happy for my classmates as I was for myself. I had not done anything; *we* had.

Reflection

We do our best work when we are part of a team. Who is on your recovery team?

207.

One of the military schools I attended to prepare for Ranger School was called Airborne School. It had been designed during World War II to prepare soldiers for the paratroop divisions. Toward the end of school, we went through "jump week," in which we took the five parachute jumps to qualify for our airborne wings. These jumps took place with different sorts of parachutes at different altitudes so that we would have some familiarity with the conditions we would experience in the Army's paratroop units.

As a young person going through this training, I did not make much of the later jumps. The one that stood out most was the first. There is a moment when you are told the jump will begin in 30 seconds. The aircraft's door is open so that there is a 180-mph wind howling past the doorway. You cannot hear a thing, so all the commands are done with hand signals. In the silence of extreme noise, I stood watching the young person standing at the front of the line. Beyond his shoulder I could see the door to a 1,200-foot drop. When the jump instructor motioned for him to go, he stepped out into the air without hesitation. I rushed behind him with the other students, none of us hesitating when it was our time to step out of the aircraft because of the example set by the young person before us.

Reflection

One of the most perfect forms of service is the one we provide with our example. The next time you are in public, remember that there is someone watching you to know what it is like to live sober.

208.

I have reflected on the fact that I will never know the young person who led us out the door on my first military parachute jump. I never saw his face. I will never know where he came from, what his life had been like. He will live his life without knowing that I will never forget him. He stood through the same 30 seconds I was experiencing. He was deafened by the same overwhelming noise, buffeted by the same violent wind. All of us had prepared for that moment. All of us would jump that day, but only one of us would be first. He wasn't very big or strong or special; it was just his turn to remind the rest of us what courage looks like. When he did, it wasn't with a grand gesture. He simply did what he said he would do, in the way his people needed. He comes to my mind often to remind me that honor is mostly humble and ordinary; he reminds me of the simple beauty of keeping your word.

We are all him—a young person waiting at the door, stepping out into space when it is our time to do our duty. We are more than our fear.

Reflection

We do not need an endless supply of examples when it comes to virtue. We just need a few good ones, people whose behavior lifted our heart. People whose behavior reminded us of who we are. We do not need many examples of honor, but we need to cherish the ones we have. Who has been an example of virtue for you?

209.

When great things are beginning, we do not yet have the skills or the resources we will need to complete them. The life we have been living is still crumbling away around us even as we take our first steps toward the new one. Success seems unlikely, but a sense of the importance of our undertaking pushes us forward. We are often very alone, but we do not feel alone. In some fundamental way, we are rejoining the human race. We walk into a 12-step meeting, or step onto our mat, or take our seat on a meditation cushion in an effort to understand ourselves.

It is a moment that changes all the moments that will come after it. It is a choice that reflects all the choices that have come before it. It is an act that gives voice to the prayers held in the hearts of our ancestors as they labored toward a better world for their children. We do not do this alone. We never have. Each step of the way has been paved by the efforts of those who came before us. Each step we take is in the name of future generations. We may have been alone in our addiction; we are never alone in our recovery.

Reflection

I find it helpful to reflect on how people have worked to give me the opportunities I enjoy. I find it helpful to reflect on how my efforts are creating opportunities for the next person who needs help. I find it helpful to remember my place under the stars. You may too.

210.

I took my seat at my first meditation retreat in an effort to accomplish something I knew nothing about. I wanted to be a better teacher. I wanted to be a better father. I wanted to be a better husband. I wanted to be a better friend. I wanted to be a better person. I wanted to be of service. There was so much I wanted. Wanting got me up in the morning. Wanting pushed me to do my very best, day after day. Wanting got me to attend a meditation retreat. But wanting could take me no further. Wanting could not give me what I wanted.

As if this were not tricky enough to understand, the reason I wanted so badly was that I did not know who I was. My meditation teachers were going to have to address the fact that I had lived in ignorance of my true nature. But before they could do that, they would have to teach me to how sit still.

Reflection

Three thousand years ago the great teacher Lao-Tzu wrote that "the path forward seems to go back." To get what we want, we have to stop wanting. To do that, we have to learn how to sit still and listen. Are there groups of people around you who have undertaken the training precept of refraining from the use of intoxicants? Do these groups offer a chance to sit still and listen?

211.

During my first few retreats, my mind raced. It wasn't meditation's fault. My mind had been racing for quite some time. Sitting in silence tends to reveal whatever is going on around you. If there are birds singing outside, sitting in silence helps you listen to them. If the air is cool in the morning or if the sun is warm in the afternoon, sitting in silence helps you feel the level of warmth. Spending time in silence helps you tune in to the world around you. The same is true when it comes to what is going on inside you. I would sit still in silence in an effort to find peace, but what I found instead was truth. My emotions tended to run hot and cold. I would be up, then I would be down, then I would be up again. My mind moved a lot. Sometimes it was just a low-grade ramble. Other times it was a full-scale rant against an injustice, a betrayal, or a failure. My mind was upset about things that I did and things that I did not do. Sitting in silence revealed the depth of the difficulty I was having with myself.

Every time my mind reacted to something, my body would get tense and want to move as well. My mind would start moving; soon after, my body would too. Sitting still felt like an impossible burden. But I kept trying. One day a teacher suggested that I let go of trying. She said to let go of resisting anything. Just sit comfortably without any resistance in your body. *Let go of your resistance to being still. Just allow your body to find its natural stillness.* As my body found its stillness, my mind did as well.

Reflection

Sit still and feel if there is any resistance in your body. As you let it go, feel yourself enter the present moment. Feel the mind settle.

212.

As I was learning to let go of resistance on my meditation cushion, I was learning to let go of resistance in my teaching. I had thought that I was supposed to get better at teaching physical technique. The teachers who were succeeding around me were inventing styles of yoga. Some were putting together sequences of poses; others were putting together systems of alignment. I wanted to be better, so I did what I could to master sequencing and alignment. I thought a lot about how you could combine these two schools of thought. I thought about sequences that also taught physical alignment. It was a good idea—for someone else.

My children wanted to go to a pool in Las Vegas where you go down a slide through a shark tank. At a silent auction for my children's elementary school, my wife and I bought two nights at the hotel with the shark tank. To pay for the trip, I taught a workshop at a Las Vegas studio. Early in that class, I let go. I let go of trying to be smart with my sequencing. I let go of trying to be smart with my alignment instruction. I let go of trying. Without the extra effort, I was able to rest in exactly what I wanted to say. One minute I was teaching what I was born to teach around, through, and over everything everybody else was teaching. The next moment I was teaching what I was born to teach. Walking around a softly lit room in Las Vegas, I became the teacher I was meant to be.

Reflection

Who do think you would be if you stopped trying to be somebody?

213.

People often ask me what to teach on this or that occasion, or to this or that population. I tell them to teach the most important thing. You may work with someone only once; there are no guarantees that any teacher will get a second chance to help someone rise to the challenge of a human life. Teach the most important thing. When I stopped trying to teach like other teachers, I found I had the time, the energy, the opportunity to teach the most important thing.

I choose the phrase "the most important thing" because it is completely subjective. The most important thing will look very different from teacher to teacher, offering students the diversity of viewpoints one finds in a healthy community. The most important thing will also look very different to the same teacher from year to year, giving her the space she needs to teach what she needs to learn. That day in Las Vegas, without any conscious effort, I started teaching what my heart wanted me to teach. No more, no less.

Reflection

If you were a teacher, what would you teach?

214.

It took me three or four years to learn to sit still. It was a useful process. My mind moved from one stuck place to another, wanting here but not wanting there. My body hurt here, itched there. I wished, I hoped, I resented. I was human. I saw how we suffer. I saw how difficult it is to carry the human karma.

It began with a subtle shift. I stopped expecting myself to be better. I stopped being disappointed. I stopped blaming. This opened a door. When I stepped through it, I became an adult. When I stepped through it, I became a teacher. When I stepped through it, fear lost its grip on me. I placed my hand on the knob, I turned the knob, I stepped through the door marked forgiveness. As I learned to forgive myself, I learned to sit still.

Reflection

If we stop blaming ourselves, we can stop blaming everyone else.

215.

Learning to sit still was a lot like someone in a 12-step program going through her inventory process. It was thorough. My whole life passed before my eyes many times. I sat through hours upon hours of regret, hours upon hours of remorse, hours upon hours of resentment—the three *R*s of addiction. I became someone who could sit with the pain of life. I could accept it. I could feel the sorrow of it without needing to blame someone. This might be my greatest human accomplishment, the willingness to feel life's sorrow. Without the ability to open our heart to life's pain, we cannot serve its beauty.

Sobriety was my first step into this ability. Sitting in meetings, I felt the pain of other addicts. I was feeling their pain without needing to fix it. Knowing that all that was being asked was to bear witness, to listen as someone told her story. On my yoga mat, my empathy broadened to encompass the trauma held in my body. Just as someone learns to sit and listen in a meeting, I learned to breathe and feel on my mat. This process came full circle on my meditation cushion as I listened to my own stories without needing to fix them. When my mind moved, my body became empty of the impulse to change or do anything. Sitting quietly doing nothing, I became empty of the impulse to change or do anything about the fact that my heart holds a human life.

Reflection

We are learning to open our heart to all of it. This "opening to all of it" begins when we put down our substance; it begins, but it does not end.

216.

My path of service taught me that I cannot give what I do not have. Once the dust settled and I had mastered a rudimentary sort of competence, I was able to see what people really needed help with. The people who came to classes had food and shelter. Most of them were gainfully employed. Many had loving families to go home to each night. They did not need my help in these areas, as important as they are. Once I had figured out how to get a class from point A to point B, I saw that people needed help with their relationship to themselves. When they moved, it was a struggle. When they tried to be still, it was worse. It was not long before I knew that this was what I wanted to help people with. The struggle they had with doing the most basic tasks was a reflection of the struggle they were having in their most basic relationship, the one they were having with themselves.

Unfortunately, I was a recovering addict who had put first things first. I had learned to be sober, then to pay my bills, then to find meaningful work. These were the priorities of my first 5 to 10 years of recovery. I had sucked it up when it came to the fact that I was just like my students, with a mind that was constantly moving and a body following along like a dinghy tied to a yacht. Sitting in the stillness that comes when we learn to forgive, I found that it was not my relationship with myself that was the problem. It wasn't that I didn't like myself or forgive myself; it was that I did not know myself.

Reflection

When we move from thinking to feeling, we leave the self of the mind behind. Try it: Listen to the wind through the trees. Notice that you are present but the self isn't. Without the self, who are you?

217.

I have lived two lives in two dimensions. In the first, I was a separate self who lived ensnared in the collective karma of self, gender, race, class, time, and place. My hopes and dreams were predicated on a self given to me by a society that is oppressive at best—utterly, self-destructively delusional at worst. In the second, I am pure awareness that holds life in much the way that the sky holds the weather.

When I relax out of the suffering of this first existence into the spaciousness of the second, my body changes. The intense suffering of the first dimension simply does not exist in the second. The collective nightmare of our history demands an enormous price in the first dimension. We carry the mental, emotional, spiritual, and physical burden of a species that does not know who it is or what it wants. As we relax into stillness, this weight falls off our shoulders. I carry the burden of our collective delusion in my lower back, so this is where I feel it first when I enter the present moment. As I relax into stillness, the chronic gripping in my lower back becomes spaciousness. This spaciousness then spreads throughout my body until it connects with the spaciousness of the eternal present. In the space of a breath or two, I am no longer defined by humanity's troubled relationship with itself. I am defined by my awareness. Within this shift lies the ability to abandon suffering.

Reflection

Think of the pain in your body as something you are carrying on behalf of everybody else. The only problem is that by carrying this burden, you are making it harder for everybody else to drop theirs. When you put yours down, everybody breathes a sigh of relief. Try lying down, getting still, and relaxing. Feel your pain leave your body.

218.

My 40s were spent observing the struggle my students were having with themselves, then going on meditation retreats to observe the struggle I was having with myself. Yes, there were many days when I wondered if I had missed the boat, when I thought I had started too late and was doomed to a mediocre practice as part of a larger mediocre existence. But on the whole, I felt that I would rather be learning what I was learning too late than not at all. It was also a great honor to be a part of my meditation community. The teachers, the students, and the teachings were world class. Bringing what I could back to my yoga community seemed to help people. What's more, my kids were growing into fine human beings. It wasn't bad.

Fortunately I am a verb, not a noun. I learned to sit still, I learned to forgive, I learned to look directly at the nature of awareness, I learned to look directly at the nature of positive and negative mind states; I learned to rest in my true nature. It was all necessary if I was going to be of service. It was all made possible because when I needed help, someone was there. When I think about teaching, my heart leaps because I know I will have a chance to pass it on.

Reflection

On the path of recovery, we get what we need so that we will have it for the next person. Do what you can each day to pass it on.

219.

I am learning to rest in stillness. When things happen, I am learning to respond with love. It's a simple lifestyle, resting in stillness, responding with love. This basic formula has made my path of service all that I could hope it to be. I experience my work with unalloyed joy. My role in my family is very specific. I do not need to be special or accomplish much. My family just wants me to love them with all my heart. They would also like very much for me to be impressed when they do something special and accomplish things.

There is a stillness to it all. I am here to be loving, that is all. Everything else is just getting from place to place and cleaning the dishes.

Reflection

Resting in stillness, responding with love. Everything else is how we learn to do this.

220.

I believe we are in a new chapter of evolution. Up until now, a species would change its form, but its outlook and priorities would remain the same. The new form would just get it done a little better. When I reflect on the transformation of my outlook since rehab, I cannot help but feel that this is a type of evolution in which the form stays the same but the nature of the individual changes.

Resting in stillness, I have an experience of myself that utterly belies the self-centered outlook of ordinary consciousness. In ordinary consciousness, my needs are paramount. Life is reduced to getting what I want and avoiding what I don't want. Resting in stillness, life is the eternal moment revealing itself in all of its subtle poetry. From this vantage point, I am able to see the self-defeating chaos of the separate self. It might work for a clam to reduce life to getting what it wants, but for humans, with our enormous mental power, to turn life into a quest for gratification is doom itself. We must evolve. This is the underlying urgency of a path of service. It starts with kindness and matures into wisdom, a wisdom that opens the door to our next chapter.

Reflection

The fact that we are participating in a form of evolution is not subtle. Reflect on your change in outlook since entering recovery.

Through kindness and wisdom, we open a door for those who come behind us. For many recovering addicts, the reason to open the door is that no one was there to open it for us. We know first-hand the pain of a closed door. This pain gives us the energy we need to do what we have to do. It gives us fire and humility when we need them and constancy when only constancy will do. Our pain does more than motivate us; it gives us insight into the nature of the problem that must be solved. Our experience of the problem gives us insight into the nature of the solution. Living through each stage of a process so personal gives us a special joy when someone succeeds.

Sometimes we open doors for others who have suffered; at other times, we open doors so that someone will never know the pain we have felt. This is a special sort of service because those who receive it will never know what they have been given. My son walks through life with a special sort of smile. He is a boy who knows that his father loves him unconditionally. He knows that he will be protected, that he will be hugged, that he will be listened to. He expects to be challenged to do his best every day. He expects himself to live with honor. He has the smile of someone who knows what love is.

Reflection

One of the gifts of recovery is that we can create love instead of waiting for it to happen. Where in the life that you have now is there the possibility to create love?

222.

Through kindness and wisdom, we open a door for those who come behind us. For many recovering addicts, the reason to open the door is that someone opened it for us. Their example was completely compelling to us. There was an energy they brought to life, a moral clarity, a sense of humor, a humble dignity that we can only hope to emulate. Following in their footsteps feels like all that we can hope for. This a particularly fortunate form of karma because it means that we will be grateful each step of the way. We will give a full effort in the little moments because we know what is required in the big ones. When we are called upon, we will put our best foot forward. When we succeed, we will be gracious. If we fail, we will not quit.

My first yoga teachers gave themselves to the beauty of the process with humble sincerity. The passion they brought to serving their students was completely unambiguous. When it was my time to become a teacher, I harbored no questions concerning the level of effort to put forth. I was walking in the footsteps of truly excellent human beings who had seen something in yoga worth the devotion of their lives. When it was my time to lead students, I did so with the ease of someone who knows what he is trying to accomplish. My purpose as I walked through the door of my first class was clear: to offer others what had been offered to me.

Reflection

Who has opened a door for you?

223.

Through kindness and wisdom, we open a door for those who come behind us. For many recovering addicts, the reason they open the door is a sense of civic duty. Their recovery has given them eyes to see the suffering all around them and the energy to do something about it. Oftentimes it is as simple as stepping forward to coach a soccer team; other times, it can be running for public office.

When I was first getting sober, the AIDS epidemic was still raging in Boston. Many of the members of my 12-step community either volunteered to work in organizations that were serving people living with HIV or took jobs in those same organizations. I bicycled in the Boston-to-New York AIDS ride in its first two years; in the second year, my future wife and I rode together, having raised $5,000. I cannot fully express in words how grateful I am that my first spiritual community responded the way it did to a community in crisis. Their response opened a door to compassion for me.

Reflection

Be the change you want to see in the world.

224.

We cannot turn back the clock. We cannot have a better childhood. We cannot relive the years we lost to addiction. We cannot undo what was done to us or by us. What matters is what we do now.

The promises in the first book ever written on 12-step recovery are said to come true only if we are painstaking in our recovery. According to Bill W. in the *Big Book*:

> We are going to know a new freedom and a new happiness. We will not regret the past nor wish to shut the door on it. We will comprehend the word serenity and we will know peace. No matter how far down the scale we have gone, we will see how our experience can benefit others. That feeling of uselessness and self-pity will disappear. We will lose interest in selfish things and gain interest in our fellows. Self-seeking will slip away. Our whole attitude and outlook on life will change. Fear of people and economic insecurity will leave us. We will intuitively know how to handle situations which used to baffle us. We will suddenly realize that God is doing for us what we could not do for ourselves.

Reflection

These are promises.

Chapter Six

Effort

The effort we put into our recovery is similar to someone walking in the forest who has determined that the deer paths, which offer easy travel, actually lead nowhere. Having learned that it is unwise to continue walking the paths she has traveled, she undertakes the hard work of creating her own path. A part of her effort moving forward will be devoted to abstaining from the well-worn paths to nowhere; another part of her effort will be devoted to blazing a new trail. She will need a lot of energy. The work will be relentless. She must be as well. With each day that she abstains from walking the old deer trails, they become more overgrown, offering her less and less of a temptation. With each day that she walks her new trails, they become increasingly smooth and wide.

In this section we will look closely at the role effort plays in the spiritual traditions that can support your recovery.

225.

There have been a few moments in my life when insight just showed up. In those moments, my life didn't change; I did. One of those moments happened when a friend offered me my first job as a yoga teacher. Suddenly I knew that it was important that I teach yoga. I'd had a similar moment 10 years before, in the middle of Ranger School. On that day I understood the role effort plays in making our dreams come true.

I had been training for four weeks; I would be training for over seven weeks more. Throughout that first month, we hardly slept or ate, nor did we bathe. But during a rare administrative pause in our training schedule, we were allowed to shower and sleep in beds. It would have been a big deal if we weren't numb with fatigue. I found myself alone in a bathroom looking at myself in the mirror. The training was similar to a meditation retreat in that my inner dialogue had essentially stopped. I looked at myself for the first time in a month. The inner quiet that had settled over me during the training allowed me to see myself without judgment. I was simply looking.

As I looked, I knew what was necessary to complete my training. I was in the middle of the most important challenge of my life, and I knew how I would succeed. I had entered the training with the same confusion that every Ranger student has. Will I make it? What I knew looking at myself in the mirror was that it wasn't a question of making it or not making it. It was a question of stopping or not stopping. I knew that what I had learned would certainly get me through Ranger School, but I had a larger insight about life in general.

Looking, just looking, I knew that we could dream anything, begin anything, but whether or not we would achieve anything would come down to this: Would we quit or would we keep going? I knew that night that the big things in life happen to the people whose effort outlives their challenges.

Reflection

For the addict, recovery is the big game. We want something intense, something important to be a part of. Well, here it is. Will you quit or will you keep going? Will your effort outlive your challenges?

226.

The Buddha called it wise effort, Patanjali called it burning zeal, and Bill Wilson called it vigorous action. None of them appear to have been confused about what they were asking of us. They felt it was important to spell out the kind of effort we needed to put into our survival because somewhere along the road to civilization we had forgotten.

A few years back, the BBC created an award-winning documentary that captured nature in all of its infinite beauty. One weekend, while I was teaching in Cleveland, my hosts entertained me with this documentary on a spectacularly large, clear television. The aerial shots of enormous flocks of flamingoes were perhaps the most beautiful images in this magnificent work of art, but two scenes stood out to me as examples of what we have forgotten when it comes to effort.

In the first, a snow leopard carries a dead mountain goat in her jaws up a sheer cliff to her cubs. It is an impossible task but she never sways in her determination. Each time she fails, she picks up the massive goat in her jaws to begin again. It is the most profound demonstration of commitment I have ever seen. In the next scene, a gigantic shark almost has a very small seal in its jaws. The two battle, with the seal using the force of the shark's attacks to fly above its jaws. The experience must have been 100 percent terrifying for the seal. The desire to give up, simply to be free of the horror and tension, would be overwhelming to a human, but the seal never stops fighting to survive.

Reflection

Others can tell us how to survive the disease of addiction, but all of the effort will come from us. But you already know that.

227.

It may be natural for a leopard or a seal to fight for survival, but addicts have lost the knack. We are the quitters who believe our quitting is a political statement. We are the adrenaline junkies who think their contempt for life is a form of bravery. We are the spiritually bankrupt whom Bill Wilson described as having lost all that makes life worthwhile. It is not easy to get the average person to leave her comfort zone. For the traumatized addict to be willing to work hard enough to save her own life requires nothing short of a miracle.

Fortunately, miracles happen pretty much as often as needed. In the book *A Course in Miracles*, scribed by Helen Schucman, a miracle is defined as a change in perspective. In this course, you pray to be willing to see things differently. In the addict's course, we crash and burn to see things differently. It's as if we drink, drug, crash, and burn our way into a new perspective on purpose. We simply will not be satisfied until the way we have been living is no longer possible. Redirecting that energy toward positive, life-affirming behaviors is no small task. It requires clear steps to take, a well-worn path leading to well-being, and the willingness to walk it. If those factors are in place, all that is required is the right sort of effort. An effort that is steady, an effort that is for rather than against, an effort that will outlast the challenges it was meant to overcome.

Reflection

We have been the destroyer, and now we must learn to be the creator. Make a list of the differences.

228.

In the rarefied air of advanced meditation studies, we learn that the energy we will put into our recovery is entirely neutral. We can put this energy into chasing a drink or we can put this energy into chasing recovery. The energy does not care. This is why I find inspiration from almost any form of mastery. The concentration of the gymnast is the same as the concentration of the brain surgeon. The effort each has made to get to the point where they can perform at a high level is the same. The purpose of the effort is different, but the skill that goes into refining the effort is the same. In that vein, I thought I would share a short list of practices I associate with those who have learned to sustain a high level of effort.

1. They train with others who share the same aspirations.

2. They stay grateful.

3. Their aspiration is to uplift.

Reflection

Review the list. Write it down on a piece of paper and keep it in your purse or wallet. Take it out in a year and see what has happened.

229.

Two stories:

Mark Hall was a highly touted wrestler who lost his first college match in front of 16,000 fans cheering wildly for his opponent. After he lost, he said the stadium was so loud with cheers for the victor that he could not hear himself think until he was in his locker room. When asked what he learned from that experience, he said that he had learned to be grateful for the size of the crowd. He said they were there to see wrestling. He said he had learned to let their love of his sport inspire him to put his best foot forward. He went on from that match to win a national championship in front of 19,000 fans.

Kelly Slater, the greatest competitive surfer in history, took a few years off at the height of his career to work on his inner life. He came back expecting to regain his place at the top of his field. It would be four difficult years before that happened. He came close several times and endured countless setbacks. Eventually he would regain his world title 5 more times for a record total of 11. When asked about his ability to keep going through the hard years, he said, "Losing is where you learn about yourself. Losing is where the good stuff happens inside. You don't go out to do the thing you're best at because you want to beat somebody. You go out and do the thing you're good at to make people better."

Reflection

Why do you put your best foot forward?

230.

Mark Hall and Kelly Slater have had an enormous impact on my life because of the way they approach learning. They did not come back from an addiction, but their quest is the same: How can I make the most of today? How can I live today so that I will have more skill tomorrow? Their dedication to learning is written in bold strokes, making it easy for others to learn from their example. They have sought out others who share their aspirations, have stayed grateful, and have been motivated by the desire to lift others up. Their walk through this lifetime demonstrates some concrete steps we can take.

When Mark Hall was in eighth grade, he was invited to spend his summer at the Olympic Training Center in Colorado Springs, Colorado. He was spending his school year far from home so that he could be on the best high school wrestling team in the country. Saying yes to this offer meant spending even more time away from his family at an early age. It was an Olympic year, so when he showed up it was in the midst of the most intense training cycle in his sport. That first summer was unforgiving, but he has never looked back. Every summer since then, instead of taking some time off like the rest of his generation, Mark has endured more intense training cycles than the one he takes on during the school year. When he is interviewed about his schedule, he expresses gratitude for the opportunity to learn from the best. He does not appear to enjoy the grueling work any more than anyone else would. What makes Mark special is that he does not begrudge it. He does not seem to mind paying the price for getting what he wants in life.

Reflection

Mark Hall's attitude toward hard work teaches us what it means to live life on life's terms. Can you free yourself from the impulse to begrudge the price life is asking for the life you want?

231.

To live life on life's terms, with the sort of grace that is implied by that 12-step term, is a spiritual skill the Buddhists call *upekkha*. It is the last of the heart qualities our ancestors cultivated as they learned to embrace their humanity. The English translation for *upekkha* is "equanimity." My teachers explained it as "not making a burden of our duties." Mark Hall does not make a burden of his duties. He does not need to pretend that training hard all winter then training hard all summer while competing at the highest levels of his sport is easy. But he recognizes that it is the price he must pay to live the life that he wants to live. More than that, he is grateful for the opportunity.

Reflection

If we are grateful, our duties will not be a burden.

232.

To meet the duties in our life without making a burden out of them frees up the energy we need to turn them into opportunities for learning, service, and kindness. What makes Mark Hall's accomplishment so impressive to me is that he achieved it at such an early age under the most strenuous circumstances imaginable. If this ability hinged on physical gifts, one could just say that it was easier for Mark than for most people. But equanimity is not a function of physical ability or circumstances; rather, it is a result of our worldview.

Stephen Covey wrote that successful people begin with the end in mind, which is to say that we know why we are doing something before we do it. Equanimity happens when we stay connected to why we are doing something as it unfolds. Through all the fluctuations between pleasant and unpleasant, we stay connected to why we are engaged in a process. We keep our eyes on the prize. This perspective enables us to stay grateful and steady as we trudge the road to a happy destiny.

Reflection

Knowing why we are doing something before we do it and staying connected to our original intention as the process unfolds is a skill in action. When we connect to purpose, we meet life on life's terms. What helps you connect to purpose?

233.

Kelly Slater became the most important person in his profession by the time he was 20 years old. The next six years were spent in arduous, high-stress conditions. He was struggling with a self-admittedly unformed sense of himself while trying to beat the best surfers in the world day after day, year after year. It was a difficult existence. We in recovery can learn from some of the steps he took to make his life more manageable.

The first thing he did was study his sport in detail. He did a fearless and thorough inventory. For a number of years, he scrutinized the scoring sheets from his competitions to learn about himself. He became self-supporting so that there would be less drama in his life. Paddling out in the midst of a stressful moment, he realized if he focused on his breath and took it one stroke at a time, his mind steadied. By taking it one stroke at a time, he lost touch with his problems and reconnected to his life. Once he learned to steady his mind, he began to look at the connection between his state of mind and the results he was getting in the water and in his life.

Reflection

The key ingredient in Kelly's success was his willingness to take responsibility for his life. He never felt perfect; he was just willing to start where he was and do what he could. What would be a good place for you to start?

234.

There is a self-sustaining quality to the type of effort we need in recovery. We need to go to meetings often enough to enjoy going to meetings. When we do, we will find our lives forming around getting to meetings. We need to meditate often enough to enjoy meditating. When we do, we will find our life forming around getting to our meditation cushion. We need to practice yoga often enough that we enjoy the practice of yoga. If we do, we will find our life forming around getting to our mats. We need to serve others often enough that we forget that there was ever any other way to be in the world. When we do, we will find our lives forming around a path of service.

We choose a path, we walk the path, the path chooses us, we become the path.

Reflection

What path are you becoming?

235.

The effort we put forth to avoid or abandon negative behaviors is the same whether we are talking about yoga, meditation, or 12-step work. The effort to cultivate and maintain positive behaviors is also the same. Yoga and meditation have made a unique contribution to my recovery by establishing the connection between how I am being in my body and how I am being in my mind. In a 12-step program, wise effort is limited to what we do. In yoga and meditation, wise effort extends into the experience of being.

One time, a meditation teacher was having us get ready for an exercise when he said something very simple. "Sit with the quality of stillness and ease that brings the mind to stillness and ease." In that moment I understood why yoga and meditation are primarily nonverbal physical experiences. My teacher was explaining that when the body finds stillness, the mind does as well, when the body finds ease, the mind does as well. This opens the door to a nonverbal, embodied skill set in which we develop the relationship between body and mind. The fruit of this skill set is the ability to bring the mind to still clarity through wise effort.

Reflection

Get still, then begin to relax. What happens?

236.

We constantly experience the aspect of wise effort that concerns the relationship between the body and the mind. When we start to hurry, the mind starts to hurry. When we slow down, the mind slows down. When the mind starts to worry, our breath gets tight. If we counteract that contraction with a couple of deep breaths, the mind relaxes and gets less fearful. In sports we have to be in the body and the breath in just the right way or we will not be anywhere near our potential. As we become familiar with the right state of body and breath for optimal performance, we start to experience how this produces "the zone" in which time slows down and the mind becomes clear.

In any form of excellence that you can name, there is a process of entering the zone of peak performance. This involves being in the body and the breath in a certain way. If we achieve this certain way, the mind enters the zone. Because of the circumstances of peak performance, we think of the zone as a special state that only the best performers achieve with any regularity. Yoga and meditation teachers shrug and call this wise effort. They explain that wise effort is to be cultivated and maintained throughout the day. Once this habit is established, there will be time to discuss the zone.

Reflection

Sit and breathe without any resistance to sitting and breathing.

237.

At the beginning of yoga class, the self is like the sun at its height shining its light on everything. The world is a mirror reflecting the light of the self, blinding us to anything but that light. As we take our seats, the process of self-forgetting begins. As we lengthen our spine, the first shadows appear. We rest in a quiet afternoon. As our heart opens, we step into twilight. As we rest in stillness, the first stars come out. Letting go a little more, we find ourselves under a nighttime sky, the sun a forgotten memory.

As a yoga teacher, I lead people into wise effort by offering two priorities. One is to be upright with an open heart. The other is to let go. Balancing these two priorities places one's attention on the action of the body. As the mind focuses on this task, the self vanishes.

Reflection

As you are sitting, balance the two priorities by sitting both upright and relaxed. As you find the middle, notice that you have found the moment.

238.

The Yoga Sutras describe in great detail the two priorities we bring into balance to enter the present moment. The process of balancing these two priorities is wise effort. The two priorities are the intentions you are meant to hold as you attempt to understand your self and your world. The first of these priorities is *abhyasa*. It is the work we do to align and repeatedly realign our attention to the present moment. *Abhyasa* is the practice of choosing connection and learning to rest in connection.

Meditation has gotten a bad rap in yoga because people find *abhyasa* difficult at first. However, a lot of things are difficult at first. The problem does not lie in *abhyasa*'s inherent difficulty or in people's ability to meditate. It lies in the habit of choosing connection and trying to control connection. We may have come by this habit honestly after a few millennia of bad results from out-of-control situations, but the skill of *abhyasa* is learning to be present without needing to control the process. As a recovering addict, I have found this skill to have a broad range of applications.

Reflection

Sit still or lie down with your attention on the rise and fall of your breathing. Practice being with the process of breathing without trying to control the process of breathing. Let the breath breathe you.

239.

It often takes years, but eventually we figure out what our teachers are telling us about *abhyasa*. We are learning to be right there without trying to control being right there. It is a subtle form of effort that we are learning, the easiest way to learn it is to find the middle between being steady and letting go, hence the importance of wise effort. Before we understand the physical skill involved in cultivating and maintaining our connection to the present moment, we may spend years in a mental version of whack-a-mole trying to get our thoughts to stop. Once we realize that when we sit still, our mind will become still, our learning will begin in earnest.

Sitting still with as little effort as possible is the first breakthrough on the road to *abhyasa*. I tell my students to give a full effort but not an ounce of extra effort. As they learn this, I tell them to begin to include the rhythm of the breath. Resting in the stillness of the body and the rhythm of the breath moves the dial considerably. We are not worried about controlling the mind. Instead we are focused on how we are sitting and breathing. We are not trying to stop anything; we are learning to experience something.

Reflection

Moving from control to connection is a physical shift that is felt in the mind and opens the heart. Try it. Listen to the sounds of the street outside. Give a full effort but not an ounce of extra effort. Receive the experience of listening as you would the taste of soup.

240.

We are learning to rest in connection with the present moment because the human mind has developed the habit of turning away from it. Someone who has not tried to meditate could live her entire life without becoming aware of how often the mind inserts itself between her and the world around her. Like someone who has grown up in a city all her life might have no real sense of the difference between what she is used to hearing and the silence of a forest.

One could ask, "What's the problem? So the mind moves around a lot. Do you want me to stop thinking?" It's a good question. According to yoga, the problem is that the mind constructs a reality with a self in the middle in the way a bubble chart is made. In our mind, we need to decide if we should go right or go left, and we create some rudimentary imagery to help us decide which way to go. We might imagine an outcome associated with each direction and a self that would be based on the direction we take. This is not the worst way to make a decision. The problem starts when we begin thinking we are the rudimentary image the mind has made up simply to resolve a temporary dilemma.

We can observe this process by watching a sporting event we do not care about. After a short while, we begin to root for a team. To respond appropriately to this situation, the mind devises a scenario in which we are a "fan." More important, we feel actual tension during the game. We feel positive or negative emotions based on the outcome. The team wins, and the fan is happy. The team loses, and the fan is sad. Now imagine what happens if we have been a fan for several decades and how being a fan has shaped your perception of reality. You could insert a religious, political, or cultural identity here if you like. Then imagine something that has the power to wake you up from the dream of being a fan so that you can remember your true nature.

Reflection

Try it: Watch a sporting event that you do not really care about. See how quickly you become attached to one side and how that attachment becomes an identity that you have real feelings about. Then leave the room, get still, and take a breath. Observe how quickly that "reality" fades.

241.

The process of making up a self and measuring the world by how it treats that self is called *avidya* in yoga and *avijja* in Buddhism. The first *a* in *avidya* means that it is an active form of misunderstanding where we are making stuff up. If we cling to the stuff we make up, we will find ourselves seeing backward, thinking that things that will make us unhappy have the power to make us happy.

When we enter the present moment, we experience a temporary reprieve from a more or less constant state of misunderstanding. By resting in connection with the present, we have the opportunity to gain insight into the nature of the mind. We see how it turns away from the present and creates a rudimentary world whose only purpose is to solve the problems of the rudimentary self it has created. Meditators experience connection with the present moment to be liberating because the rudimentary self and its problems are stuff we make up, stuff that we can't bring with us into the present moment. When the mind becomes still, the self and its problems vanish.

Reflection

What were the problems your "self" was using during the six months before you came into recovery? What were the problems your "self" was worried about two weeks ago? How important do the problems your "self" is having feel today? How important will they be a year from now? Now sit and begin to slow and deepen your breath, feeling the breath from beginning to end. How many breaths does it take to feel better?

242.

When you consider that human suffering can be escaped by entering the present moment, you can see why our work is important. Wise effort is the skill set we develop to enter the present moment. *Abhyasa* is the first of the practices we learn as we regain our connection with the present moment. It is a faithful, steady sort of effort in which we patiently return to the felt experience of life over and over again, moment by moment, day after day, year after year. This faithful effort is practiced on our mats, on our cushions, and in every moment of every day.

The easiest way to remember to align your attention with the present moment is to notice when your mind has become particularly troublesome. Sometimes your mind will deliver stunningly powerful negative emotions, but it can be equally disquieting in its ability to steal away the ordinary moments that make up your life. Coloring with your toddler, listening to your friend as she tells you about her day, making a decision, giving a lecture, taking a bite of your lunch—you name it, the mind will find a reason to be somewhere else. Each time you feel yourself slip out of the mystery of the present and into the dreary narrative of the mind, patiently reengage the skills that you are learning in yoga and in meditation. Come back to the felt experience of the body. Come back to the felt experience of the breath. Relax back into the felt experience of life.

Reflection

Start using idle moments in your day to practice resting in connection—at the bus stop, in your bedroom, during a quiet moment at work. Spend some time in your own company resting in your connection to life.

243.

I can tell when I am practicing *abhyasa* faithfully because my outlook improves dramatically. I get a lot of the momentum I need by teaching yoga. Attending meditation retreats and following them up with a disciplined home practice works pretty well too. Spending time in nature with friends is another winner. However I do it, when I spend more time in connection than in distraction my mood elevates. My body is full of energy, my mind enjoys life's challenges, and my heart is full of joy. I find myself laughing out loud often.

Time in connection relieves me of the worries and stories, of the separate self, replacing them with the joy of being. It is a great trade. *Abhyasa* delivers the energy we need to excel on our own spiritual path. It also has the ability to connect us to the qualities of heart, mind, and body we will need on our path of service. We do not really need to get "good" at it; we just need to keep putting one foot in front of the other on the road to the present moment.

Reflection

Begin to notice which situations leave you depleted and which leave you elevated. Then see which move you more into your head and which move you more into the moment.

Once we are resting in connection with the present moment, our mind clears. Our senses heighten. When I was teaching hot yoga, I could feel the difference between 95 and 96 degrees. Our sixth sense heightens as well. As I settle into the moment, I can feel a class I am teaching at a level of understanding that is deeper than what my eyes could deliver. I can feel when my students are warmed up; I can feel when they become mentally exhausted but still have physical strength left. I can feel the mental and emotional tone in a room. I can feel a class's relationship to time; I can feel when psychological time is present and when my students have left it behind.

We open the channels to our senses when we enter the present moment, but more important, we open our channel to inspiration. While I am feeling a class warm up, I am also listening for guidance from my intuition. My intuition will come to me visually, offering a pose or a sequence. It will also come to me in a sense of which direction to take an experience in. Stepping into the present moment is like stepping into a multidimensional crossroads. The roads carry information. Some of the information comes from the five senses, some from the sixth sense, some from the collective wisdom of the class, and still more from the universal mind, the mind of infinite potential, the mind of infinite correlation. Learning to be a teacher is learning to stand at this crossroads feeling into the part we will play on that day.

Reflection

Get still and feel your senses awaken.

245.

The Yoga Sutras instruct us to abandon the mind's habitual movement in order to see clearly. It is as if we were a glass of water with sand stirred up in it. The sand is composed of the habits of the mind. The water is pure awareness. The practice of yoga allows the sand to settle so that we have access to the water's true nature. Attachment stirs things up. Aversion stirs things up. The violation of healthy ethical boundaries stirs things up. As we seek to avoid or, if necessary, abandon these habits, we cultivate habits that settle the mind. Loving-kindness is settling. Generosity is settling. Wisdom is settling. Connection is settling. Honesty is settling. Sobriety is settling. *Abhyasa* not only settles but brings us right there as life is happening so that we can observe what creates confusion and what creates clarity.

The next practice of yoga allows us to participate in life without getting lost in it. It allows us to pay attention without getting stirred up. This practice is called *vairagya*. Learning this skill is very much like a dog learning to watch squirrels run around in the backyard without chasing after them. For a dog the only reason to do this is to conform to the wishes of his pack. Our motivation in this scenario is to know what is true about the squirrels in our backyard. The backyard is our mind-body, and the squirrels are our thoughts, emotions, sensations, intuitions, and inspirations.

Reflection

The classic analogy for vairagya *is that we become the sky that holds the weather. Get still and relaxed as you feel into your breath. Then hold the experience of breathing in and breathing out like the sky holds the weather.*

246.

In *abhyasa*, we rest in connection as an unending series of thoughts, emotions, sensations, impulses, fears, regrets, fantasies, and memories land in the felt experience of our bodies. We have learned to move when there is something that we want. We have learned to move when something is threatening. We have been taught to exert control over our surroundings. Failure to do so has meant death. Now we are well into a life that has further confused the situation by offering an unending series of consequences whether we have chosen to act or not, and we are instructed to be steady, to be still, to be engaged but not to act. Rather, we are to trust and to allow.

But there is good reason to consider this instruction closely. The dog can only hope to catch enough squirrels to survive. He cannot figure out the nature of squirrels, domesticate them, or begin a small business offering better squirrels for a lower price. He was born to see squirrels, chase them, and eat them. When he stops being able to do this, he dies. The human has infinitely more options available to her than the dog does. But she must use all of her abilities if she wishes to exercise those options. The first is her ability to focus on the task at hand. The second is her ability to watch a process through to its end, to see what is true about a thought, an emotion, or an attachment.

Reflection

Begin to watch how life pulls you this way and that. Feel how not letting yourself get pulled seems harder than just living as a leaf in the wind. Pause just long enough to feel the discomfort of not acting on an impulse. Start becoming familiar with that discomfort.

247.

If aligning and repeatedly realigning our attention with the present moment is difficult, letting things play out without attempting to exert some form of control over them feels next to impossible. Itch after itch, ache after ache, we scratch, we shift, we fidget. After 10 days of not scratching for as long as we can, we end up scratching after all. We go home only to speak out intemperately. We eat the dessert after all. Disappointment and existential angst are definitely two of the hardships of spiritual practice.

As long as we are reacting internally, we will continue to react externally. The key skill is non-reaction, and it begins with a humble sort of patience. With that patience, we start reacting less intensely to the fact that we have reacted.

Reflection

The next time you react, don't be so disappointed. Try not getting angry with yourself for getting angry; try not being impatient with yourself for being impatient. Soften a little to the fact that you are human. Smile as you see that you are beginning to see.

248.

Practice allows us to take a life skill and place it in a manageable context. Instead of learning kindness at work with your abusive boss, you sit quietly offering loving thoughts to a cherished pet. I began the process of learning non-reaction within a simple specific context. It was the moment in meditation when I noticed that my mind had turned away from the present. One minute I would be doing okay, resting in connection, the next moment I would be having a political argument with people who were not there. In that moment of recognition—that moment when I had blown it again—I learned to soften.

The practice is to meet pain—our pain, our neighbor's pain, nature's pain, the world's pain—with compassion. This heart practice gives you a way to be with your mind when it wanders. It gave me a way to be with my disappointment at having failed again with my meandering mind. I have given this practice a full effort. Once I notice that my mind has wandered, I wake up, alert to the moment I am in. This is the moment of peril and promise. I can harm myself or learn to accept myself. As I breathe into acceptance, I discover a deep compassion for the struggle of being human. It is hard to have an intention that you have not yet lived up to. It is honorable to try day after day. Meeting my wandering mind in this way has taught me how to meet the people in my life who are trying day after day.

Reflection

How do you treat the people around you who are trying day after day? This is how you are treating yourself. Practice allows you to learn how to treat yourself better in just the smallest steps at a time. One way to begin is with the moment you take a bite of something you like to eat. This is a moment for learning kindness. Go a little slower and let the pleasant nature of the experience grow into joy.

249.

Once I began softening my attitude toward my drifting mind, I saw the importance of this moment. The way we react to the wandering mind is the way we react when something or someone disappoints us. Instead of the habitual surge of aversion, I was learning to soften into compassion. This opened the door to understanding. Aversion narrows our vision; compassion broadens and deepens it.

Softening into compassion gave me some room to maneuver. I could look at what the mind had been up to and what it had been like to be stuck in that particular loop. What had triggered the pattern? Who was I when I was caught in this loop? Was I a victim? A villain? Was I willing to feel how hard it was to be human stuck in my loops of repetitive thinking? Could I be gentle? Could I have faith? Could I go back once more to the effort to cultivate my connection to the truth?

Reflection

Recovery is the choice to treat yourself better. What small steps can you take in your recovery today to be gentle when you disappoint yourself?

250.

"Still the body, still the mind, still the voice inside;
in silence, feel the stillness move."

— KABIR

With practice, we become less and less disturbed when the mind wanders. When we notice that the mind has gone off somewhere, we soften to bring it back as simply as we would adjust our laces before tying our shoes. No surge of emotion, just awareness and a subtle action taken. This allows the mind to settle. The combination of *abhyasa* and *vairagya* practiced over time produces an increasingly quiet mind that can begin to observe what happens when it is still.

Our dog is resting quietly. He has learned to use the body and the breath to bring the mind into a restful state. He has developed the emotional steadiness that is called equanimity. The impulses caused by the running squirrels do not bother him that much. By combining restful ease with equanimity, our dog has practiced into a new possibility. The running squirrels are no longer food in the dog's yard. They are aspects of the larger tapestry of life—movement, stillness, sound, and silence.

Reflection

When our personal hell becomes the disease of addiction, we are able to look at it differently. What had been personal is now a part of the larger tapestry of life teaching us what it is like to be human. What is it like to sit quietly as other people speak in such a way that you are learning to comprehend life?

251.

We can think of ourselves as developing two complementary skills, focus and allowing. To understand how these two abilities are simultaneously practiced, it helps to think of them as intentions. One intention is to be right there as life is happening; the other intention is to allow life to unfold. "To be right there as life is unfolding" means that the two intentions are pouring themselves into one experience.

Reflection

As we progress in our practice, we begin to think in terms of balancing complementary opposites like discipline and freedom. Recovery balances an honest appraisal of our challenges with a profound faith in our ability to overcome them. What are two opposite priorities that you are learning to balance today?

252.

The settling process of yoga and meditation reveals the presence of awareness. As we look directly at the nature of awareness, we discover the ability to balance *abhyasa* and *vairagya*. We are not a body or a mental construct like a "self" or a "me." We are an aware presence. This awareness holds the experience of the body the way the sky holds the weather. If you sit still, you can watch how awareness holds the sounds of the street outside in the same way it holds the sensations in your body. Awareness is equally "out there" holding street sounds and "in here" holding the sensations of the breath. If we relax a little more, we can actually bring the experience of awareness into our awareness.

When we collect awareness around something specific, we call it focus. When we rest in non-attached appreciation, we call it spacious allowing. In *abhyasa*, awareness is focused attention; in *vairagya*, awareness is spacious allowing. Both experiences are effortless expressions of awareness. In meditation, we learn to work with the different properties of awareness, combining them as the moment demands to achieve connection and understanding. Sometimes more focus is needed; at other times we need more spaciousness. The truth is always found in the middle.

Reflection

Sit still and listen. Move between focus and spacious allowing. Listen to something specific and then pull back to listen to the world around you. Move back and forth. Then look at what's listening.

Internal Expression of Wise Effort

Wise effort is expressed in terms that are both internal and external. There is the external concept of an honest effort, or a full effort in which we learn how to put our best foot forward. Then there is the internal expression whose domain is the relationship between the body and the mind. We have talked at length about an honest effort. The final essays in our section on wise effort will be dedicated to the internal expression of wise effort.

253.

To explain the skills of yoga to new teachers, I use the story of Galileo and how he used a set of lenses to observe the movement of the stars, leading to a number of insights about the size and shape of the earth. The Yogi is using her skills in much the way Galileo used his lenses. For her work, the Yogi has three primary lenses: kindness, concentration, and non-attachment. Each of the primary lenses has a number of secondary lenses. For example, under kindness, you will find non-harming, compassion, joy, and equanimity. By combining these primary and secondary lenses properly, the Yogi is able to see with remarkable clarity into the nature of her own experience. This subtle action is wise effort.

Once we have learned the art of wise effort, we are able to look deeply into the nature of looking itself. We see how we are not really seeing at all. Rather, we are labeling things and reacting to our labels. By combining kindness, concentration, and non-attachment, we are able to see that the labeling process belongs to the part of our mind that creates images in an attempt to understand the world. These images are accompanied by thoughts that create stories. The images and stories move together to create a temporary self in a temporary reality in an effort to gain a temporary benefit. This swirl of images and stories gives us a glimpse of why the Yogis felt there had to be a benefit in seeing without all the mental movement. At this point we begin to practice in earnest. But unlike Galileo, whose focus was on the stars, ours is on the space between them.

Reflection

Pick one of our three primary skills: kindness, concentration, or non-attachment. See how bringing it into a moment changes the way you are seeing.

254.

"We see the world not as it is but as we are."

— ANAÏS NIN

When Galileo adjusted the lens of his telescope, he changed what he was able to see. The Yogi has no lens; instead, she is adjusting her mental states to be able to see more clearly. She begins by adjusting her physical state to bring her mind into calm, clear connection with the present moment. This attunement of the physical body is a verb, not a noun; it is a continual process of refinement. Like a tightrope walker, there is no moment when she stops balancing. As she learns to balance her body in a way that stills the mind, she becomes able to feel the difference between the mind in contracted movement and the mind in connected stillness.

Watching the mind shift back and forth from stillness to movement gives you a chance to feel your emotional reactions to both states. If you are anything like me, you will start to become attached to stillness and averse to the chaos of mind-made images and stories. These emotional reactions become a new form of suffering. Your quest for non-attachment will yield a new attachment. A period of denial, frustration, and suffering will ensue, but you will eventually develop a new lens, self-compassion. You will decide to be kind to yourself as you watch the mind doing what it has done for thousands of years.

Reflection

Feel the difference. Bring your gaze to one point and feel your mind become quiet. Then let your mind move back into its habitual thinking. Do it several times. Which state feels better? Now try being kind to yourself as you attempt to bring a little more stillness into your days.

255.

Balancing the body in a way that brings stillness to the mind begins the process of self-inquiry. From the experience of a still, spacious mind, we are able to understand the nature of a moving, busy mind. Watching closely over time, we are able to see how everything is connected and happening more or less at the same time. Our mental movement is accompanied by an emotional reaction, which is accompanied by a physical reaction. If we move our body in a hurried manner, we start to experience an anxiety that makes it hard to think straight. As this understanding deepens, we see how the skills of yoga can affect our experience. How a posture is a state of mind. How kindness is a state of mind. The way a slow, deep breath changes our point of view.

Observing cause and effect as it relates to our mental, emotional, and physical experiences explains the role practice plays in improving our quality of life. If we practice skillful states of body, mind, and heart, we will feel them at every level of our being. It is not long after we learn to enter the present moment through the body that we discover the power of loving-kindness.

Reflection

Think of someone you love. What happens physically, mentally, emotionally? Think of someone who disturbs you. What happens? What do you think would happen if you focused more on those you love than on those who disturb you? This is called practice.

256.

One of the turning points in my recovery came when I first heard the phrase "The way we see the problem is the problem." My sobriety had instilled in me a passion for living wisely. I loved behaviors that made sense. Going to meetings made sense. Paying my bills on time made sense. Being kind to the people in my life made sense. Finding a way to share what I was learning in recovery made sense. Yoga did not exactly make sense. How was a triangle pose in yoga any different from a bench press in the gym? I went to the gym because it made me feel better in a number of ways. I went to yoga because it made me feel better in a number of ways. I knew there was a difference, but I could not put my finger on it.

In *The 7 Habits of Highly Effective People*, Stephen Covey's statement that "the way we see the problem is the problem" turned on a light. I had known for some time that cathartic exercise wasn't the point of yoga, but I did not know how to start thinking about what the actual point was. Covey helped me to see that yoga could teach me to understand how I was seeing the problem. By entering the same poses day after day, I could watch my mental habits. I also saw another possibility. By entering the same poses day after day, I could practice new ways of seeing. What if this pose was not a means to an end? What if this pose was not a performance? What if more was not better? How would it change my experience if I had faith, or patience, or joy, or focus? In meetings I was learning new things to do. In yoga I began learning new ways of being.

Reflection

In anger I see a slow waitress. In kindness I see a young person trying to be responsible for herself and learning a difficult job. Begin to study the relationship between what you are feeling and what you seeing.

257.

I spent the next 20 years learning how I was seeing the problem was the problem. Some of the time was spent trying to change my mind about things. At other times I learned strategies for doing so, such as taking space or journaling. My approach during these times was essentially external. I would do different things to see differently. There are skillful actions in yoga, but they are described as the external disciplines. Yoga encompasses a set of internal disciplines as well. The confusion I often felt during these years of my learning curve was the result of trying to accomplish something with an external discipline that could only be accomplished by an internal one.

Buddhist meditation teachers taught me the internal skills of yoga. Once I started sitting on meditation retreats with the Buddhists, I began to see how to participate in a yoga pose in a way that allowed me to examine how I was seeing. The patient attention I was learning on my meditation cushion taught me how to be patient with myself as I experimented with my attitude and outlook on a yoga mat. The work I was doing on my mat joined with the work I was doing on my cushion, offering me a place to really understand how I routinely participated in life. Watching how I participated in a pose or a meditation gave me a chance to feel into the underlying beliefs and assumptions that drive my behavior. I had found a place to learn how to see how I was seeing.

Reflection

Name a behavior that changes your perspective. Now name a belief that does the same.

Positive and Negative Mind States

Combining time on my mat with time on my cushion has given me a list of positive and negative mind states that I can feel affecting my point of view.

Daily Reflections on Addiction, Yoga, and Getting Well

258.

Gratitude

Early in my recovery, I discovered the link between my frame of mind and the quality of my life. At the time I had a legion of negative states of mind but just one positive one. My early recovery tool bag of healthy mind states consisted of one tool, gratitude.

Still quite young, I became familiar with the spectrum of human emotion that can be captured in a single word. When I prayed, when I sat in a meeting, or when I went to bed sober, resting for a moment on clean sheets, I would feel the peace of a sober life, a peace that filled me with gratitude. It was a new experience to be deeply touched by life. I had felt gratitude for getting something, but the depth of feeling that filled me during those first years of sobriety was something entirely new. Listening to the wind through trees at night or considering what my 12-step community was doing for people touched my heart in a way that I had never experienced before. I saw the beauty of life. I felt the eternal, exquisite, heartbreaking beauty of life. Sometimes tears would come, but usually it was too big even for tears. I felt the sacredness of the living. I felt sacredness in stillness, in silence, in the willingness to try. I saw the beauty in vulnerability, the dignity of courage, the sweetness of love. In a moment I would feel it all. In a moment I would see why. Pierced by life's unspeakable beauty, I would know that gratitude is the place to stand, the song to sing, the love to give.

Reflection

The positive psychology movement suggests that people partner with a spiritual friend and email them one thing they are grateful for once a day for 21 days. Try it.

259.

Proving

I have always enjoyed sports. Growing up, I loved everything about them. Sports were the only thing I did well enough to make my mother smile. As I grew older, sports became the only thing that I did well enough to make myself smile. As addiction trashed the rest of my life, I could still prove my worth on a wrestling mat. For a number of desperate years, I clung to the self-respect I could claim because of athletic achievement. It was an empty form of self-respect, but it was all I had. I fought hard for it. I learned the habit of proving. Proving to the world and to myself that I had the right to live at all.

As a sober person, I abandoned the athlete's pride for the recovering addict's humility. But the habit of proving hadn't gone away. It showed up in my desire to be the best—the best waiter, the best EMT, the best counselor, the best teacher, the best Yogi. Not some existential best, but rather the best in the room. Better than my peers. Better than my co-workers. Better than my friends. Trying to be the best on my mat hurt. Trying to be the best on my meditation cushion was absurd. For a number of difficult years, I unlearned the habit of proving myself in everything I did. I felt the sadness of the pain I had caused in relationships. I felt the pain I had caused myself. I felt the pain of living lost in a delusion. I learned the skill of self-compassion. I became gentle when my mind wandered or my body ached. I became kind to myself as I tried to learn about a life without winning and losing, a life with nothing to prove.

Reflection

What if there were nothing to prove?

260.

Being Steady

As an addict, I did not value my word. I quit, I cheated, I lied. I enjoyed it when someone in a movie acted with honor, but I felt no kinship. I belonged to the lost tribe of the honorless. Attending 12-step meetings gave me the chance to act honorably. I would stay until the end of the meeting to pick up chairs. When someone needed a sponsor, I would raise my hand. To the best of my ability, I lived the values and the principles of the program that was saving my life. When it was time for me to be a part of the yoga community, I did what I could to participate with honor. The same was true when I found a meditation community. To this day, how I show up to these communities means more to me than what I get from them.

One of the features of honor that I have learned by attending yoga trainings and meditation retreats is how to finish something. Finishing with honor places a process in a position to lift up whatever we do afterward. As we look back, we remember that we kept faith until the last breath of the last moment of what we said we would do. There is a temptation to get the "goods" from an experience and bolt before the awkward process of closure, the final, vulnerable moments of goodbye. Being honorable has meant, among other things, learning to be steady and willing to feel the discomfort that accompanies the end of things. I have felt a special joy as I have watched my children embody this skill. Steady as they show up for the first day of school. Steady as they go through the process of the school year. Steady as they get ready for graduation. Steady as they pose for pictures holding flowers given to them by proud family members. Steady as they finish with honor.

Reflection

Watch for the tension that arises toward the end of things. Feel the desire to bolt. Really feel it come, change, and go. Being steady means that we are able to access our intention regardless of what is going on inside or outside of us.

261.

Comparison

Is thinking it would be easier if we were someone else

Better if we were someone else

Is thinking that if our circumstances were different

If we could have more time

More money

More opportunity

Different challenges

It would be better

Comparison is never having what you need to succeed

Reflection

The next time you compare yourself with someone else, ask yourself how that feels. What are you doing to yourself when you compare?

262.

Contentment

During my first year in recovery, I learned the practice of "blooming where you are planted." Take the energy you have freed up by being sober and build a life right here, right now. Don't waste any time wishing things were different. See the opportunity in the life that you have now. Yogis believe we must be content to start with the body that we have, the health that we have, and the mind that we have. We must learn to start where we are.

Spiritual communities are formed to get work done. They are a place to make important changes. When groups of people gather in this fashion, they learn to work with what they have.

Reflection

Feel the difference. Consider the possibility that you will need things you do not have yet to succeed. Then consider the possibility that you can start now, with what you have now, and get wherever you want to go in life.

263.

Faith

I lived for 26 years in a world without faith. My world did not contain faith the way deserts do not contain whales. What I had was fear and the courage to face it. Courage was all that mattered. We could die in fear or die with dignity. Courage was the only thing I had, the only thing that could not be taken away. There was a time in my life when I longed for war so that I could express my disdain for fear and death. I had nothing worth having, but I could die without fear, and that was something.

Then a power greater than myself lifted my addiction. Healed by grace, I found myself among people who were choosing life unconditionally. It was too beautiful. It was utterly unforeseen. One moment I was a child preparing for death, the next I was a young person surrounded by love and possibility. My heart swelled with a new faith in life, faith in my fellow human beings, faith in the process of recovery. I found that what lies beyond fear or courage is the humble, enduring strength of faith.

Reflection

Write down a list of things or people in which you have faith. What is it like to have faith?

264.

Judgment

I am told all living beings share the survival strategy of creating separations. To say this is good and that is bad, or this is yours and that is mine. Humanity with its supercomputer of a brain has taken this survival strategy and turned it into a form of suffering. We say this way that I am is good, or this way that I am is bad. This way that *you* are is good, or this way that *you* are is bad. Or these people are good, and these people are bad. We measure the world in the way we measure ourselves.

Being steady in our practice reveals the painfully limiting effect this has on us. It is as if our true nature is to be a river, and each time we judge, we contract into a pond. Being a pond is hard when being a river is our destiny. The pain of it forces us to look at the habit of judgment. Is it possible for life to flow through us without contracting? Can we know the truth of something without judgment or labels? Can we be like a river, letting life flow through us without resistance?

Reflection

Judgment is the story we are creating around a feeling. The discipline is to shift our attention from the story to the feeling it is trying to manage. What can you learn from the feeling beneath the story?

265.

Trust

Any actual step forward is a leap of faith. If we take enough of them, we come into what is called verified faith, a faith that has been confirmed by experience. At this point we are no longer taking leaps of faith; we are taking leaps of trust. As addicts, we have broken faith, broken hearts, and broken trust. Before that, our own hearts were broken in ways that were so unbearable that relief was all that we could hope for. Living in the darkness of an endless winter, we sometimes remember the colors of flowers, the warmth of the sun on our skin, the smell of summer grass cooling as the sun sets. Walking into a meeting for the first time is not an act of faith or trust; it is an act of despair. After a few weeks, it becomes an act of desperation. But on the day I received my three-month chip, the desperation gave way to something sweeter.

The August sun was still fairly high in the sky as I walked into an evening meeting in Frankfurt, Germany. My sponsor was there, as were my counselors and the gentleman who had taken me to my first meeting. I felt young, healthy, and hopeful. My long winter was ending. The colors of spring were returning to my heart. I could feel a faith forming in me that one day would be trust.

Reflection

If trust feels like too big of an ask, start with willingness. Let your duty be the willingness to try. Let your leaps be ones of willingness.

266.

Ill Will

I have been mistreated. I don't like it. I have contracted around my dislike for certain moments in my life, certain situations, certain people. I have felt real pain that has caused real patterns of behavior. I am human. Yoga could be described as learning what it means to be human. To do this, we learn to become still so that we can feel. Resting in what it feels like to be human, we discover that however natural it is to harbor ill will toward those who have harmed us, might have harmed us, or may harm us in the future, the experience of this natural inclination ranges from unpleasant to a sort of inner hell on earth. Ill will simply is not worth it.

But the logic of ill will feels impenetrable. "She harmed me. I don't like her at all. When I think of her, it makes me so upset!" Keeping score paints us into a corner. This is why self-compassion is such an important part of one's recovery; without it, there often does not seem to be a logical way forward. Self-compassion is the voice that says, "I can't go on like this. Yeah, I know she did this and I did that, but I'm done drinking poison and hoping someone else gets sick."

Reflection

Redemption does not mean having a different past; it means becoming whole. Self-compassion is the belief that we deserve to be whole.

267.

Interpersonal Goodwill

Deepak Chopra wrote that we can access spirit with the question "How can I be helpful?" I gave this teaching an honest effort and found it to be true. "How can I be helpful?" feels like the secret to success for anyone who is working as part of a team. Whenever I ask this question, I move into a posture of service to a situation I have chosen to be in. I am expressing a willingness to place whatever abilities I possess at the disposal of my fellow human beings. For a moment in time, I am no longer talking about goodwill. I am being it.

To practice a skillful mental state like goodwill, we need to put forth two forms of effort. The first is the effort to cultivate goodwill. We choose to let go of other ways of being as we begin to manifest goodwill in every aspect of our being. Goodwill informs our physical body, our energy body, our emotional body, and our mental body, and our channel to divine goodwill opens as well. The second form of effort we need to put forth is the effort to maintain. Once we are in the posture of goodwill, we need to rest in it. We need to fully receive the experience of goodwill. As I have worked to understand this second effort, I have learned that the surest way to maintain a state is not to work at it but to become it. The second effort is to be the change we want to see in the world. Having chosen goodwill, we step further out of the way in order to be it.

Reflection

For the next week, find opportunities to ask how you can be helpful, and feel the difference. Feel what it is like to choose goodwill.

268.

Goodwill as Citizenship

I was talking to a class recently about the quality of heart we call goodwill. I said kindness is what we feel toward a puppy. Goodwill is what we feel toward a community. They are two very different felt experiences. When I am being kind to my children, I am in a primal flow of affection. There is no complexity, only an intense form of love whose physical expression is kindness. When faced with the complexities of a relationship to a community, it may take a while for this sort of feeling to arise. Goodwill, on the other hand, does not depend on the recipient being furry, small, and cute with big eyes. Goodwill flows from the purity of our heart's intention. As such, goodwill is not a response to something outside of ourselves; rather, it is a statement concerning what lies within us.

The victory of goodwill is that we are not content to let the world dictate our response to it. Goodwill represents our ability to choose from the truth of our heart rather than from the relative truth of our judgments. This provides a twofold service to our community. We are acting for the highest good while demonstrating the ultimate form of human freedom, the ability to choose how we respond.

Reflection

In goodwill we discover a profound freedom—the freedom from circumstances.

Daily Reflections on Addiction, Yoga, and Getting Well

269.

Enthusiasm

A coach I very much respect was talking about his athletes' preparation for a major event. He talked about why he felt they were preparing well. He said they were focusing on their effort rather than on any results they'd had so far or any results they were hoping for in the future. He said they were having fun, which made them enthusiastic as they made the most of the opportunities that were available to them. He stopped at that point to clarify: "You have to be enthusiastic, right? Without enthusiasm, you aren't much good to yourself or anyone else." This was an arresting moment for me. The coach in question is one of the most successful people I have ever seen. He also tends to keep his cards close to his chest in interviews. The fact that he stopped to elaborate on enthusiasm in such specific terms revealed how important it was to him. I felt like I had been given a precious gift. This man who had successfully dedicated his life to excellence could not help but pause to give respect to the role enthusiasm plays in the work we do and the victories we achieve.

I reflected on the felt state of enthusiasm. How does enthusiasm feel? When do students regularly move into this state? Then I thought back to the interview: "They are having fun."

Reflection

The next time you are with friends having fun, feel how "having fun" generates enthusiasm for whatever the moment brings. Then consider the mental state of enthusiasm. Is there any task that is not made easier if we are in a state of enthusiasm?

270.

Wise Effort

Wise effort is central to the success of someone on the path of recovery from addiction. At its most basic level, it refers to the quality of effort that freedom demands. This effort has four applications:

1. The effort to avoid unskillful states of mind

2. The effort to abandon them once we get caught in them

3. The effort to cultivate skillful states of mind

4. The effort to maintain skillful states of mind

The unskillful states of mind are pretty straightforward: greed, hatred, and delusion. A skillful mind state is any state of mind that does not create suffering. An example of a skillful state of mind is gratitude. Another is connection to the present moment. Once a person understands that recovery is her primary purpose, she quickly realizes that using happens after she has been caught in an unskillful state of mind. She may not realize it, but her "program of recovery" is essentially her method for enacting the four forms of wise effort in her life.

The subtlest aspect of wise effort is its ability to bring the mind to still clarity. We enter the present moment through the body and the breath using the meditative application of wise effort. We come into this form of effort by finding the middle ground between steadiness and ease, stillness and rhythm, steadfastness and letting go. As the body finds the middle, the mind finds the moment.

Reflection

A program of recovery is a plan to cultivate skillful mind states while avoiding or abandoning unskillful ones. In particular, what states of mind lead us toward our substance and what states of mind lead us toward recovery? A good day is when we spend more time in positive mind states than in negative ones. What is your plan for having a good day?

Chapter Seven

Mindfulness

This chapter will explore how mindfulness heals our relationship to the support that exists all around us all the time.

271.

People in recovery have chosen to believe that there is a way of life available to them. For a while, this belief is all we have. However, before too long we find ourselves in the presence of people who believe as we believe but have done so for a longer period of time. These people have not only found hope; they have found a plan. This book is dedicated to sharing the essence of three of the "plans" I have found. All of them are very optimistic. It is an article of faith in yoga that to those who seek, the divine is near. The Buddha taught that the ultimate truth is close at hand calling out to be seen, to be known. Bill Wilson wrote that once we become willing, "the door opens almost of itself, and looking through it, we shall see a pathway." The premise of mindfulness is extremely positive. It states that what we are seeking is already at hand; we just need to open our eyes to see it.

Reflection

Let yourself feel into the idea that humanity is very close to the answers it seeks about its own existence. Imagine that your recovery is part of humanity's movement toward these answers. Then imagine that what is called for is the willingness to see what is right in front of you without commentary or embellishment. This is mindfulness.

272.

Eckhart Tolle's teachings did not make sense to me until I began to consciously connect with the present moment. Once my meditation practice had given me a sense of how the present moment felt, his teachings concerning awareness without thought became extremely helpful. One of his statements that I found very helpful is that we see the world through a screen of beliefs, labels, and judgments. Mindfulness is the ability to see without this screen.

The training of mindfulness has two basic components. One is the ability to keep the mind rooted in the present. The second is described as "bare attention," the ability to see without Eckhart's screen. This training can begin in a 12-step meeting, on a yoga mat, or on a meditation cushion. We simply need to stay with something for while and come back to the same practice day after day. As this consistency takes hold, we begin to see the habits of our own mind. We start to become familiar with the way the mind wanders, and how this wandering robs us of our connection with the truth we are seeking. Perhaps for the first time, we realize that when we return from the mind's wanderings, we do not even know what we missed.

Reflection

When we are consistent in our meeting attendance, yoga practice, or meditation practice, we are given a chance to observe the habits of our mind. What practice have you made a clear commitment to?

273.

Consistency in practice is how we are able to observe the habits of the mind that cause us to suffer. Once this consistency has been established, mindfulness begins as a willingness to pay close attention. The ancient phrase translates as "to ardently watch." Sitting quietly in a meeting or on a meditation cushion, we begin to watch our reactions. Coming back to the same commitment, the same setting, the same practice allows us to become familiar with some of our most prominent mind states.

After a year or so, going to meetings began to serve this purpose for me. It was a subtle process. For a while there was the meeting and then there was my tumultuous inner life. I did not make the connection that my inner life was one of constant reaction—that I was reacting to what was happening or reacting to my thoughts about what was happening. I just knew that my experience of going to meetings tended to move back and forth between a rapturous appreciation for the beauty of what was taking place and a squirmy self-centeredness whose essence was an aching sense of lack. One minute I was in rapture, the next minute I was not getting called on even though my hand had been up for a while. One minute I was in rapture, the next minute I was wondering if the woman across the hall liked dogs, because if we were going to get married, it would suck if she didn't like dogs. I was very far from understanding the concept of skillful and unskillful mind states, but I was beginning to feel them.

Reflection

Before we begin to practice mindfulness, we tend to blame a situation for our reaction to it. We get tired of "that scene" or "those people in the meetings" when what we are actually tired of is our habitual reactions. We feel we can either bolt to a different situation or settle for a less-than-optimal setting. Mindfulness gives us a middle path.

Around my third year of going to meetings, I started to get a sense of my habitual mind states. There was Virtuous Me, who loved the meetings, loved the process, loved sobriety, loved the community. Then there was Craving Me, who wanted attention, validation, relief, control. The best craving Me could hope for was the desire for a "better" future. Virtuous Me was living a dream come true. Craving Me was so close I could taste it. A stage of my recovery was learning to accept these two versions of myself living within me. I was too new to the path to have a sense of what I could do about it. All I knew was that I really liked being virtuous, but craving spoke to me in terms I had to agree with as well. I wanted success, I wanted love, I wanted validation. That was real for me, as real as my gratitude for being sober.

Trying to be virtuous while denying the existence of craving seemed like a plan until it turned out that craving got way stronger when I met it with resistance. All my early interpersonal and professional sobriety fiascoes came from this tactic. Yoga helped a little. I could go somewhere that was quiet and private and feel how lost I was, how the struggle of being human was actually more than I could bear. Then I was taught to sit, to accept, to receive the moment. Just be still and let go. No ifs, ands, or buts. Sit with the sadness—the longing, the anger, the hope, the fear. I was told to sit with my aching heart. When I did, craving became feeling.

Reflection

The next time you are in craving, stop, relax, accept, and feel. Move from craving to feeling.

I drank to escape my inner life, even though, at the time, I might have told you I was drinking to have "fun." I think I believed that the plan was to drink and have fun. That was certainly the fantasy on the way to the liquor store. "I am going to drink, and it will be way better than if I did not. It will be pleasurable at worst, downright fun at best." That was the story, and I stuck to it. In reality I drank because my inner life was an unmanageable concoction of normal adolescent predicaments, intense unresolved ongoing trauma, and addiction. Within this nightmarish scenario was a young person trying to sort life out. Drinking laid all of that to rest. Drinking obliterated the complexities of my life in favor of a comfortable numbness.

My strategy had been to run from the truth. The antidote was to sit with it. By the time this became the plan, I was extremely ready for it. I had had more than enough of trying to manage the unmanageable. I am amazed that I did not die at some point from my utter lack of interest in trying to addict my way through life. The pain of avoiding life gathers in us like a snowball rolling downhill. This pain begins to lessen the moment we begin to think about facing life honorably. Sitting down with intention to be still, to accept, and to receive the truth of life as it is right now sets another ball in motion, but instead of gathering suffering, it will gather wisdom. It will gather freedom. It is a large concept, a large experience, this thing called freedom, but you can hear its call in the distance the moment you stop running and start sitting.

Reflection

Try sitting still and letting yourself be stillness. When you are still, what do you hear?

276.

The movement from craving to feeling has been a work in progress. Putting down the drink helped, but the momentum of my old life carried on for some time in recovery. I managed my craving by going to meetings, going to work, drinking coffee, eating sugar, and having drama.

Stepping onto a yoga mat changed the course of my recovery. My teachers created a place where I could learn how to feel. I felt the in breath; I felt the out breath; I felt where I was holding tension in my body, I learned to soften. I felt my feet, I felt my hips, I felt my hands. I learned to feel how I was sitting. I learned to feel how I was standing. I learned to feel how I was lying down. I learned to have an intimate relationship with the taste of my food. I learned to feel the water brushing my feet at the edge of a lake. When I looked out over a silent forest valley, I could feel my own heart and all the hearts that had been touched by the beautiful mystery we call nature. Yoga taught me silence, safety, and intimacy. I felt so much that I started to feel when I was in craving and when I was not.

Reflection

It might help to think of yoga practice as a way to feel back into life.

277.

I will be forever grateful for the depth of feeling that yoga has helped me to access. But it was not enough to fundamentally change my point of view. My addict story did not end when I got sober. Everything I experienced during my first decade of recovery was organized within the distorting construct of my story. This included the experiences I was having on my mat. There were moments of peace and clarity, but it never occurred to me that I could experience life outside of my story.

This was the problem I encountered when my daughter was born. My wife looked at me and told me in so many words, "This is not going to happen within your story. You are going to have to open up your point of view to include entirely different ways of seeing things." Up until that point, if I experienced something, I would write it into my story. From that point on, I had to find a way to stop being the author and start being the learner.

Reflection

It helps to see what happens when you take a couple of breaths that are slow and deep. Breathe in a way that you can feel the breath from beginning to end. Breathe in a way that you can feel the spaces in between. What happens to your story when you breathe that way? What happens to the main character?

Sobriety gave me a chance to feel, yoga taught me how to feel, and meditation taught me how to relate to what I was feeling. Mindfulness is how I learned to have a feeling without making up a self or a story to go with it. It began with my wife needing me to be able to see things differently and my inability to do so. This caused such a crisis in our lives that I started going on meditation retreats. I did not really know what I was getting into or why it would be helpful, but I knew I needed to do something and that it would be peaceful.

In the beginning, I attempted a sort of mindfulness without wise effort. I really wanted to be "right there" for the in breath and the out breath. I would tense up and concentrate on the breath then get angry, frustrated, or disappointed when my mind wandered. This felt like the best I could do: trying too hard, failing, becoming frustrated, and then repeating. At some point during these meditations, my body would start hurting and I would struggle with my body in much the same way I had been struggling with my mind. I was taking the whole thing very personally, which is great when you are succeeding, but my efforts were being met with very little success. At the end of the retreats, however, something would change. In spite of it all, I would leave with a profound enthusiasm for meditation. I made every effort to follow up my time on retreat with regular time on my cushion at home. Things kept getting better. It was not that I started to take the process on my cushion less personally; it was that I was taking less person to my cushion. Without knowing it, I had begun to forget the self as I embraced the moment.

Reflection

Mindfulness is learning how to have an experience without a story or a self, just the experience. Start small and listen to the sounds outside, or taste each bite of food. How does it feel to listen without inner commentary? How does it feel to taste without inner commentary?

279.

To prepare for these essays, I am reviewing writings on mindfulness. I sit and read the same lines each day, letting them connect to my own experience of sitting in meditation. One of the qualities of mindfulness is that it is an absolute refusal to leave the present moment, regardless of what the present holds. We are being taught an unwavering commitment to the truth. We are being taught that the truth is happening now. We are being taught that the truth needs us. We are not receiving the truth that the moment holds merely for ourselves; we are receiving the truth on behalf of all beings. It is through us that life experiences the truth.

You can feel this in the rooms where people sit for days in silence. You can feel how we are meant to dedicate our lives to the truth that is revealed when our minds become still. You can feel how the choice that is being made is to place one's life in the service of life itself. In perfect paradox, this movement in personal and universal consciousness begins in stillness. In perfect paradox, we start by learning how to stop.

Reflection

The mind turns away to make up a truth. Mindfulness says, "No, the truth is already here." Relax, breathe, and feel the truth that is already here.

280.

The Yoga Sutras have a term, *citta vritti*, that refers to the habits of the mind. The word *vritti* means "turning." At the beginning of our practice, the habit of the mind is to turn away from the present moment in order to think about what just happened. Mindfulness is a retraining of the mind. In mindfulness we are learning to turn toward the present moment in order to understand it. This turning toward the present moment is easier said than done.

For thousands of years, humans have differentiated themselves from other species by being willing to stop and think before they acted. This has given us a tremendous advantage over creatures that have wanted to eat us and creatures that we have wanted to eat. We can plan ahead, reflect on past experiences, and anticipate in ways that nothing else in nature appears to be able to do. By turning away from what is happening and turning toward our thoughts, we have devised an infinite well of creative responses to life's challenges. This has been so successful that we appear to have only one channel, the thinking channel. Mindfulness has proved its ability to bring this situation into balance. By learning how to turn toward the moment, we become free to think or not to think as the situation demands. This becomes particularly important if our thinking is causing suffering.

Reflection

A simple exercise is to count breaths, counting 10 breaths and then counting back to 1. Notice what happens to your body when your mind turns toward the breath and rests in connection. Notice what happens to your body when the mind turns away and starts to move into thinking. Feeling the difference is how you connect to the truth.

281.

In many situations, the human capacity for thought offers us a tremendous advantage. We can take abilities that many creatures demonstrate, like preparing for the winter or building a shelter, and turn those abilities into a civilization, an economy, an art form, or a city. These same abilities can also make us endlessly miserable. Everything we encounter becomes an occasion for more thinking, thinking about a self we are making up as we go along. Thinking about a self that does not have what it needs or has what it does not want. Thinking about a self that makes us unhappy when we think about it. As if this weren't bad enough, we measure the world in terms of how it impacts this character that we are making up as we go along. To get a sense of the problematic nature of measuring the world by our "self," imagine if we understood everything in terms of how it impacted dog shows, or spin classes, or the taste of tomato soup. "Will moving our society in this direction improve or lessen the taste of tomato soup? The answer to that question will decide my vote."

Measuring the world by something as completely arbitrary and temporary as the "self" does not make any sense, which is why human history looks the way it does and why individuals throughout history have believed there has to be a better way. We've tried a number of strategies to offset human self-absorption. We have created political, economic, and religious paradigms to address our tendency to think our way into suffering. Mindfulness challenges us to look directly at the moment to see the role the mind is playing in our relationship with life. What happens to our perspective when the mind is thinking? What happens to our perspective when the mind is calm and clear? What can be done to turn the mind toward the truth?

Reflection

A simple exercise is to watch the habit of measuring the world by your "self." See if you can catch yourself evaluating a situation in terms of what you would have done or how it might affect your "self." Are you in truth, or are you having a physical and emotional reaction to how you imagine the situation will impact your "self"?

282.

After a couple of years of regular mindfulness meditation, I began to understand the term *settling*. A few days into a meditation retreat, my teachers would say that we were becoming settled. I often did not feel settled, nor could I notice anything particularly settled about the people around me. While sitting during shorter, less arduous meditation once I was home, I would notice a change in my mind that took place. I would sometimes begin a meditation on a bad note. Fighting against my mind's desire to be thinking would seem hopeless for a while, but then suddenly I would be in calm peace, with my breath a slow rhythm, my mind clear, awake, spacious.

Mindfulness is a commitment to a process. This particular process is a form of paying attention. We place our attention on one of our five senses and keep it there, patiently returning the mind each time it wanders. This will settle the mind over the course of a half-hour meditation or over several days on a meditation retreat. The implications of settling are worth examining. Getting stirred up is a process. Settling is a process. It means that we can choose which process to practice.

Reflection

A simple exercise is to spend time in silence. No talking, no reading, no writing, no screen time—just silence. Your mind might rebel at first, but if you stay with it, before long you will be seeing the world with a mind that has settled.

283.

Learning to settle the mind is not a small thing. It requires us to learn how to sit, let go, forgive, and feel. It requires us to be patient and kind with ourselves. When these factors start to come together, we develop a familiarity with the mind in connection with the present moment—how the mind becomes silent like the silence around us, still like the stillness around us, with clear awareness like the clear awareness around us. We experience a mind that is an aware presence; it has no self, just as the sky has no self. We begin to understand the Yoga Sutras and the teachings of the Buddha. We begin to understand what it means to be empty, for the habits of the mind to cease. We see why these things are part of our spiritual evolution. We see why they are part of how we come into contact with the truth.

As I became familiar with the experience of a settled mind, my perspective on life began to change. Perhaps the most important change was how I understood happiness. With a settled mind, I see that I exist in an eternally perfect moment. I see the utter wholeness of eternity, how nothing is lacking. The logic of craving, which drives much of our public and economic life, no longer makes sense to me because it is based on the belief that in this time and this place, there is something lacking. The hope of craving is that at some point in the future, if we get what we want or get rid of what we don't want, we will be happy. Resting in the clarity of a settled mind, I saw that true happiness must be found in the present moment or it will not be found at all. The trap of suffering is looking elsewhere for what is already here.

Reflection

A simple exercise is to lie down and become perfectly still. Relax, breathe, feel. What is lacking?

284.

I began turning toward the present moment in earnest while I was leading a yoga studio in Manhattan. The world around me could not have been less still. There were millions of people within a couple of miles of me at all times. Within Union Square, you could see thousands of people day and night. Thousands. The Whole Foods store across the park had three floors. The Barnes & Noble next door had four. Human beings were trying to get somewhere all around me all of time as I was slowly embracing the idea of being here.

One of the ways that I learned to create some space within all of this manic activity was to do one thing at a time. If I was walking the 25 blocks from Grand Central Terminal to my studio, I would not be on the phone or listening to music. I just walked. When I sat in a cab, I just sat. If I was crossing the park to lunch, I just walked, breathing in the air, feeling the temperature on my skin. To develop mindfulness is to develop one's capacity for intimacy with one's own experience. As we develop this intimacy, we discover how nourishing pretty much anything can be if we take the time to feel the fullness of it. Sitting in the corner of a coffee shop feeling my feet on the floor, the movement of the breath in my chest, I would take the first sip of my coffee and experience an exquisite privacy in the midst of thousands of people. As the taste filled me with happiness, I felt myself falling in love with the simple beauty that mindfulness was teaching me, the beauty of being here.

In the years since then, I have been grateful to have started out amid the endless sounds and sensations of New York because I am not troubled by the rattle of an air conditioner, the hum of a fan, or the sounds of traffic outside. Mindfulness is not a situation; it is a choice.

Reflection

Pick a couple of moments in your day to do one thing at a time. Maybe a walk or a drive. No music, no phone calls, just take a walk or drive. If you are cleaning or cooking, just clean or cook. Doing one thing at a time creates a space in your life for the moment to arrive.

285.

While I was running the yoga studio in Manhattan, my family was living in a carriage house in Tarrytown, New York, a 300-year-old river town on the Hudson, 30 minutes by express train from Grand Central Terminal. The upper floor of our house was one large room that served as a play area, living room, kitchen, and dining room. The lower floor was the same footprint divided into one normal-size bedroom and two of the smallest bedrooms ever made. My son was still in a crib, so he got the smallest room; my daughter got the other small room, which we compensated for by installing a rainbow awning over her bed.

Though cozy, the carriage house did not afford me a practice room. When I was not doing one thing at a time in downtown Manhattan, I was practicing yoga and meditation in my son's narrow, crib-filled room while he crawled about upstairs, making an occasional break for the gated stairs. I was turning toward the present in earnest, but the present held very little resemblance to a meditation center. It was loud and cramped, albeit love-filled. I learned to teach yoga as subway trains rumbled underfoot. I learned to meditate as Elmo squeaked overhead. I learned that turning toward the present was turning toward the present.

Reflection

When we try to exclude things from our awareness, they become obstacles. When we include them, they become the backdrop as the mind settles.

286.

Teaching mindfulness to adults feels a lot like what I imagine teaching health class to middle-school children must be like. There's a lot of squirming around uncomfortably as the class is dragged into a topic that feels awkward and overwhelming.

This is tremendously ironic because the actual experience of mindfulness relieves us of the burden of thinking problematic thoughts all the time. The energetic uplift is twofold. Mindfulness brings us out of the taxing experience of endless thinking and teaches us how to use our energy more efficiently. Each time we rest in the felt experience of the body, we are refreshed at every level of our being. Spending regular time in the present moment not only conserves the energy we would have used thinking and reacting, but teaches us how and when to use our energy. We discover that the biggest energy drain in our lives consists of negative mind states. Practicing mindfulness develops a highly attuned sensitivity to when thinking is draining us. As this sensitivity grows, we are simultaneously cultivating the ability to rest in connection to the present. One could say that we are learning to put forth the effort to avoid negative mind states while cultivating positive mind states. One could even say that this type of effort is wise.

Reflection

Imagine if humanity could learn to think only when it needed to. What if your recovery was a part of that shift?

287.

I am still learning to practice mindfulness all day. At first I just practiced it on my cushion and then went back to endless thinking. Eventually I understood what mindfulness is and saw how I could choose it as I attended to the tasks of my daily life. I understood that I could drive across town thinking draining thoughts, or I could drive across town practicing mindfulness. In time, I learned that driving across town practicing mindfulness was more enjoyable. As an addict in recovery, the choice between an unpleasant experience and a pleasant one is not really a choice at all.

I do not try to practice mindfulness all day. I break my day up into intentional moments, then practice mindfulness one moment at a time. A moment can be driving, cleaning, exercising, meditating, standing in line at the airport, or having lunch. I do not need my moments to be special. Each moment is a chance to make a commitment to resting in the felt experience of the breath as I allow my mind to settle. Moving through my day like this is peaceful and fun. Living like this places my energy in the service of my well-being and the tasks that I am performing. The alternative is to allow my own energy to be used against me. I have tried both. It feels wise to put forth the effort to use my energy to create the peace and joy of connection.

Reflection

In 12-step programs, we are taught to live one day at a time. Zen has been described as doing one thing at a time. It feels wise to live one day at time doing one thing at a time.

288.

Once I began practicing mindfulness throughout the day, the role of my meditation practice made more sense to me. Before that, it felt problematic to taste a better connection to life for a half hour a day, only to abandon it until I found my way back to my cushion. What was meditation supposed to be doing? Was it a moment of temporary relief in the midst of a life that felt like wearing shoes that were too tight? Once I saw that the skills I was practicing on my cushion were meant to be practiced throughout the day, my time spent in meditation became an actual practice.

Sitting quietly allows me to practice resting in the felt experience of the body so that when I am going about my day, I have a well-traveled path to walk on from my mind into the moment. Sitting quietly allows me to practice resting in the felt experience of the breath so that when I am going about my day, I have a well-traveled path to walk on from my mind into the moment. Each time I turn toward the present moment, I get a little more familiar with the path from my mind to the moment; I understand the ease of the body, the gentle rhythm of the breath, the subtle effort of will that moves me from thought to awareness.

Reflection

A spiritual practice like 12-step, yoga, or meditation offers us principles to live by and an intentional space in which to practice them before we try them out in everyday life. This is the connection between practice and everyday life. Take a principle, practice it, live it. Then practice it and live it again.

289.

Practicing mindfulness on my cushion and in my life has made me familiar with my mind. One of the striking realizations of this process is that I am not the metaphysical phenomenon projected by my brain, which I call "my mind." I cannot be my mind for a number of reasons. The first is that I am the one watching it. The second is that it literally has a mind of its own. If I were my mind, I would not have to practice yoga in order to train it. If I were my mind, I would choose to have only thoughts that led to happiness. I would spend days on Big Sur resting in the purest inner silence just for fun. I might forget to think entirely. Who needs to think when we can rest in the eternal now?

I am not my mind. It exists in much the same way my feet exist. My feet are a process with a purpose. When I wanted my body to run a marathon, I trained it to run long distances. With patient persistence, I partnered with my body to change what was possible. My body had been one way; I trained it to be another way. Mindfulness is similar to training for a marathon, only in this training we are training the brain through the medium of the mind. The mind has been one way, the way that was meant to keep us alive and reproducing. Now we want it to be another way. We want it to keep us connected, compassionate, and wise.

Reflection

Living one day at a time, doing one thing at a time offers us a unique opportunity. We can invest all our energies in the present moment. Mindfulness is that sort of investment. The return on the investment is peace and freedom.

290.

I am not my mind, which means you are not your mind. Without a practice like mindfulness, this simple fact could go unnoticed for many lifetimes of unconscious reactivity. We can live from one mind-made impulse to another and never realize a process that is no more you than you are your feet is calling the shots. The mind has a purpose like your skin has a purpose. We are not anti-mind any more than we are anti-skin. We are pro-truth. The truth is that you can watch the mind. You can train your mind. You can reflect on the mind without needing to react from it. This observing presence, this choosing presence, is *you*.

One of the profound shifts that I have been taught is to become aware of the awareness that holds the mind. When you watch the mind, you will find that sometimes it moves and sometimes it rests. It stops altogether when it wants to connect to the present moment through one of the five senses. Watching these different mind states, we have the opportunity to become aware of what is watching. I have been trained to witness the way awareness is holding the movement of the mind, how it holds the mind the way it holds a sound or a sensation. Watching a sound, a sensation, or a thought move through awareness, I begin to look directly at the nature of awareness. I have been taught to bring my awareness to awareness, to receive the experience of awareness. For a while, I reflect on the experience of awareness, and then, with no more effort than it takes to say or write the words, I move from reflecting on awareness to being it.

Reflection

Try sitting quietly listening to street sounds or forest sounds. Listen for a while, then bring your attention to the awareness that is listening. Then be the awareness.

291.

Not being the mind means that we do not have to take it personally anymore. We do not have to take its constant hope and fear personally or even seriously. The mind's cravings, imaginings, fantasies, and resentments are not our problem unless we make them our problem. This is the freedom of mindfulness; we get to reflect on the mind as opposed to reacting from it. When I let this sink in, my heart stops for a moment. This *would* be a freedom. But how do I achieve it?

My teachers are practical people. One of the methods they teach for finding freedom is to examine cause and effect. What happens right before suffering? What happens right before well-being? What are the near causes of suffering in your life? What are the near causes of well-being in your life? Some near causes are specific to an individual, while others are universal. One of the universal chains of cause and effect is that mindfulness is the near cause of mindfulness. Each moment we turn toward the present moment makes the next one easier.

Reflection

We can put a positive chain of events into action in our lives through commitment and practice. Choose one positive chain, such as going to meetings, sitting in meditation, or being on time to work. Commit to it and practice it. Does each time you follow through make the next time easier?

292.

When I begin a workshop, I review a basic formula with the students. I remind them that mind states give rise to behavior, then behavior gives rise to consequences. We belong to a tradition that believes if we want to experience new behaviors or new consequences, we begin by examining our habitual mind states. Our practice allows us to become familiar with the habits of our mind. Over time we develop an in-depth understanding of which mind states lead us down the road to suffering and which mind states place us on the path to freedom.

As our connection to our experience becomes increasingly subtle, we progress from knowing what anger or greed is like, to knowing what behaviors are motivated by anger or greed, to knowing what consequences arise out of behavior that's motivated by anger or greed, to knowing what the body feels before a chain of events is set in motion. Growing up in a rainy climate, I became familiar with what it felt like before rain, how that was different from what it felt like before snow, or thunder, or lightning. Repeated exposure to how the world feels right before it snows or rains gives us time to prepare, put on the right clothes, or get under cover. Meditation is like this with the habits of our mind. We begin to know when to seek cover. In time, a child knows when it is about to rain. In time, a Yogi knows if she is on the path to suffering or on the path to freedom.

Reflection

Reflect on what it is like to know something. How do you know when it is going to rain or if someone is failing to tell the whole truth?

At first a child does not know when it is going to rain. The whole thing is a mystery to her. Sometimes it rains; sometimes it does not. She may love the rain or dislike the rain, but she has no understanding of it. As the years pass, the child begins to connect the dots. She notices that when the sky looks a certain way her parents tell her to put on her raincoat. She also starts to have memories about the rain—what it is like when it comes, what it is like afterward, how the sun comes out, how it leaves puddles. The adult sitting in meditation experiences a similar process as she slowly comprehends the connection between her mind states and the quality of her life.

For the child, it does not matter that it takes a number of years to understand the rain. She possesses zero expectations concerning this understanding. However, the adult on a meditation cushion is there precisely because of her expectations. She expects meditation to effect a change in her life. She also expects to understand how this change should go. But she has forgotten how it was to learn something, how things take time. How wisdom grows like the natural thing that it is. She has forgotten, so she takes her seat to remember. She will remember the wonder of not knowing; she will remember the wonder in each small detail; she will remember the joy of learning something new in a world full of things to learn.

Reflection

The learning of recovery extends over the rest of our lives. It pays to get ahead of learning by being patient about learning. Give time time.

294.

A child knows it is about to rain from a combination of factors. To some extent, these factors can be apprehended by the five senses. The sky looks a certain way, the air begins to smell a certain way, there is an eerie calm that can be felt. These factors are considered, but the child does not want to get drenched. So she has learned to let the senses have their say while feeling inwardly for the deeper knowing that says without a doubt that drenching is imminent.

A Yogi lives in much the same way. Having been drenched in suffering, she has learned to listen inwardly for the truth beneath the story, the fear, or the desire. She has learned to be present while allowing life to flow through her. She has learned that suffering is preceded by a physical contraction, a contraction that attempts to block the flow of life itself. When the Yogi feels that she is holding on, she lets go.

Reflection

One of the understandings that yoga can give a recovering person is the knowledge of what a mind state feels like. This is helpful because mind states tend to justify themselves. Mind states make sense to us when we are in them. But if we feel beneath the story, we can know what is really going on. Begin to pause, breathe, and feel when you get caught in "stinking thinking." How does this mind state feel?

295.

After I have talked about the relationship between mind states, behaviors, and consequences with my students, I discuss the mind's propensity to turn away from the present moment. There is a basic division in terms of mind states. There are those that turn us away from the present moment and those that turn us toward it. The mind states that turn us away from the moment are described as unskillful, the ones that turn us toward the present moment are described as skillful. Unskillful mind states lead to unskillful behavior, which in turn leads to negative consequences. Skillful mind states lead to skillful behavior, which in turn leads to positive consequences.

When I am working with students for the first time, I tend to not focus that much on the mind states. I may, for example, teach them to practice with a combination of mindfulness and joy. Mind states are not ignored, but my focus is instead on drawing their attention to a specific phenomenon. I begin with exploring the mind turning away from the present moment and the effort it takes to turn the mind back toward the present moment. We look directly at the effort that is needed to turn our attention toward the present moment. As the class continues and I can feel the students starting to settle into connection with the present moment, I evoke the next form of effort. I challenge them to feel into the quality of effort that is needed to keep our attention rooted in the present.

Reflection

In some ways, our mind is a wonderful teacher. It offers us any number of opportunities to notice that we have turned our attention away from the present, prompting us to rediscover the effort needed to turn our attention toward the present. As you find yourself in meditation or as you move through your day, turn back again and again to the present moment and notice the subtle effort it takes to choose connection.

296.

Above all else, mindfulness is a skillful form of paying attention—to how the mind turns away from the present moment to create worlds of its own; how these worlds give rise to the mental states of greed, hatred, and delusion; how these mind states are a form of suffering; and how this suffering gives rise to behaviors that cause still more suffering. Paying attention to how we are *not* this process leads us to realize that we are the aware presence that is observing it.

Mindfulness also encompasses the moment when we see that we have turned away from the present moment. It includes the process of returning the attention to the present moment and the experience of the moment. Mindfulness includes the shift from observing to being. It takes it all in over and over again. Bear witness as the mind turns away from the moment to create suffering and turns back to the moment to create well-being.

Reflection

Mindfulness is the sky that holds the weather.

297.

In 1985 I went to the U.S. Army Airborne School, which is a challenging three-week training that prepares a soldier for serving in one of the Army's parachute units. I trained physically, but it was equally important to train myself mentally. To psych myself up, I would use a series of visualizations. I would see myself leaving the training, getting into my dream truck (I owned an old Chevy Nova), and driving off into the sunset. In another, I promised myself that I would go to a movie with my best friend, the comfortable joy of this vision offset the fear and discomfort of reality.

The summer after I graduated from Airborne School, I did in fact go to the movies with my best friend. The theme song of this particular movie was Tina Turner's "We Don't Need Another Hero." Sitting in the late-summer warmth at the end of the movie, I was moved to tears by the rawness the intense training had left in me, connecting me with the pathos of the song. All I had ever known was the oppression of active addiction. All I had ever known was the fight for survival. Tina Turner's words and the place they came from in her heart were something new. The acceptance, the sadness, the heartbreak that brought someone to their knees; the idea that one could acknowledge life's pain while surrendering. I was brought to tears by the willingness to be brought tears. I was brought to tears by an open heart. Silently weeping in a darkened movie theater, I felt what moves people to the practice of mindfulness. The heart demands it of us. The heart demands the truth even when it breaks, because it knows that it will be broken open.

Reflection

Sprinkled throughout my active addiction were moments when my true heart's desire could be glimpsed in the songs, movies, stories, friends, and activities I chose. Make a list of how your heart let itself be known, even in your active addiction.

298.

Active addiction appears to rob a person of all dignity, all virtue. Upon getting sober, we can only cringe at the thought of who we were and be grateful for who we could become. Mindfulness or compassion feel lifetimes away from the intention we have lived with while active in our addiction. However, this narrative does not honor the fact that we stayed alive until we could find recovery. This hit home in the starkest terms when a friend of mine who had known me from kindergarten through high school came to my house. Ned and I had not seen each other in 37 years. When we were last together, I had been deep in my addiction, so as I prepared to see him, it was with a heavy heart. I felt called to make amends for the ways that I had fallen short in our relationship. As he came through the door and met my wife, he said, "Do you know the last time I saw Rolf?" I thought, *Here goes; let the shaming begin.*

Ned then told this story: We went to different high schools playing on competing football teams. The last time he saw me, my team beat his team badly. In the midst of this drubbing, he caught a pass. I ran over to him and helped him up. As I gave him a hand up, there was a big smile on my face. With a palpable joy in his success, I congratulated him on a great catch. This is what my friend remembered about me.

When I reflect on the person in this story, it is really all I want to have been in the world. I want to have been that guy, that friend. It is not a coincidence that you chose recovery or that you are reading a book whose aim is to celebrate a life guided by the heart. That person was always there; we are simply making space for them to step out into the light.

Reflection

Our active addiction contained a number of moments when the purity of our heart's intention was revealed. Make a list of moments when you rose above your addiction to claim the virtue that you would someday live in recovery.

299.

The recovering person is choosing the light, having known only darkness. It is a process to choose the light after so long in darkness. We have to learn how to live all over again. We must learn to listen, to feel, to see. Mindfulness weaves all of these forms of understanding into a way of life that allows us to see the darkness and the light for what they are. Being a practical person, the Buddha broke things down for us. He taught that there are only three basic mistakes we make on the way to the truth: We think the impermanent is permanent; we think the unreliable is reliable; we think that which is not the self is the self. The path to the truth begins with a simple inquiry. How do these three mistakes show up in our experience of everyday life?

I started with impermanence because it is usually named first by my teachers. On my cushion, I would feel the coming and going of things. I watched how the aches and pains gave way to spacious bliss, which in turn gave way to anxiously checking my watch. In everyday life, I observed as one moment gave way to the next. The terribly uncomfortable passed. The terribly sweet passed. The interminable ended. I watched as I suffered when the unpleasant seemed to stay forever. I watched as I suffered when the pleasant left all too soon. I allowed myself to feel the pain of my expectations, hopes, and fears, as my children grew out of their sippy cups and began reading for themselves at bedtime. I let myself feel my humanity. I understood how humans struggle in a constantly vanishing world. To understand this form of suffering, I had to let myself feel the pain of it. This bore fruit. I came to understand a habit of my mind while learning something about the pain of everyone I meet.

Reflection

Watch the process of change in the world around you. Watch how you contract around it, wanting it to speed up or wanting it to slow down. Those who wish to be free and to help others live free allow themselves to feel the pain of living in a world that changes.

300.

While sitting in meditation, we observe a profound paradox. When the mind moves, the process of endless change threatens it. When the mind is still, it rests in the process of endless change as a baby rests in its mother's arms. Our problems with change begin when the mind turns away from the present moment; our problems end when it turns toward it. It is life's job to move; it is our job to be aware. Life is meant to unfold endlessly. We are meant to be awake.

When the mind moves, we invent a fictitious form of creation that stands in opposition to the actual process of creation. We say, "No, this should not be! I am the one who should dictate how all of this goes down. Life's purpose is irrelevant." When the mind is still, it is able to see the perfection of life's unfolding. The Bible describes God looking upon his creation and saying, "It is good." As I spend more time in stillness, my understanding of this passage has deepened. Each time my mind settles, I look upon creation and feel in every cell in my body that it is good.

Reflection

Sit quietly smell, feel, and see nature. What stirs in your heart?

301.

As I meditate on impermanence, I watch things come and go. As I meditate on unreliability, I watch them change. I watch the new car become a used car that becomes an old car. I observe how something that once made me happy becomes something that is making me unhappy. I observe how something that used to make me unhappy is now making me happy. Within the larger process of impermanence is the process of unreliability.

We tend to hate unreliability. We say, "In my day, this never would have happened," but what we mean is that we thought this thing was never going to change, and we feel thoroughly let down that it is not the way it used to be. We experience a few days without traffic on a certain route, but that proves to be unreliable and now there is a lot of traffic. We had a workout that was making us very happy, but now it has made us very injured. We loved ice cream, but as we get older, we learn that ice cream does not love us back. It's not that things are gone, it's that they have changed. The things we put so much faith in turn out to belong to a natural world that is in a constant state of transformation. When the mind turns away from the present, it finds itself trying to create permanence where there is none. The mind experiencing life this way is appalled. The mind resting in the present feels the stillness in the constant change. The mind experiencing life this way is enthralled. Sitting in meditation, we discover that we have a choice. We can be appalled or enthralled. It is up to us.

Reflection

When was the last time your new jeans did not become your old jeans?

302.

I was not going to inherit anything or be able to leverage anything. The only people who looked like me who received any sort of respect at all were absolutely excellent at what they did. In my heart, there is a very childlike passion to be the person who is recognized as excellent. On the one hand, this could be considered laudable. On the other hand, this could be described as an extreme form of attachment. I experience the desire to excel as both. The downside is that I have been competitive, self-centered, and unrealistic. The upside is that I have had to take responsibility for the results of my actions because it is the only way to get better at anything.

As someone who has spent his whole life trying to excel to compensate for the racial oppression I internalized as a child, I cannot recommend putting this behavior on a pedestal, but I have learned some useful ways to relate to the phenomenon of unreliability. I have been a student of people who have had measurable success in their fields; I have studied generals, athletes, writers, political and spiritual leaders. As you look closely at someone like Martin Luther King Jr., you will see that he responded to change or chaos a little better than most people do. The great ones have not had to be a lot better than the average human being. They just had to be consistent in seeing the opportunity that arises when things change. Sir Alexander Fleming, who discovered penicillin, saw the opportunity in mold. The recovering person is learning to live this way by becoming a veritable avatar of resilience. In her world, when one door closes another opens.

Reflection

The addict has no choice other than to be strong in the broken places because a broken place is where she must begin. How are you learning to see the opportunity that arises when things fall apart?

303.

We sit in meditation in an effort to understand ourselves. This effort turns out to be a process that unfolds in stages of commitment. Mindfulness constitutes the moment in our self-observation when we make the commitment to neither abandon nor coerce our experience. As we grow in our capacity for mindfulness, learning to settle into the experience of the present moment, we discover that the moment contains stillness and movement. Looking closely, we realize we are the stillness and everything else is the movement.

We are not the leaves that move in the wind. We are not the sounds that move through the silence. We are not the sensations that move through the body. We are not the thoughts that move through awareness. We are not what being cold feels like. We are not what apples taste like. We are not what love feels like. We are not what grief feels like. We are not a hope, fear, success, or failure. We are not a name or an age. We are not a race or a gender. We are not the impermanent forms of life that arise, change, and pass. We are an aware presence that is slowly coming to recognize itself for what it is.

Reflection

Try to find your "self." Can you find your self in the sounds around you? Can you find your self in sensations? Taste, smell, see. Can you find your self in the forms of life?

304.

Thinking the impermanent is permanent, thinking the unreliable is reliable, are mistakes we make then compound by making a self out of that which we are not. We make a self out of having something we don't want. We make a self out of not having something we do want. We make a self out of things not staying the same or not being the way they used to be. We make a self out of where we were born. We make a self out of who we are with. We make a self out of who we are not with. We make a self out of the language we speak, the religion we grew up with, the nature of the body we have for the moment.

Taken together, the mistakes regarding permanence, reliability, and the self create a perfect setting for attachment to arise. Caught up in a web of erroneous assumptions, we react with a roller coaster of hope and fear. Our active addiction was an attempt to manage this unmanageable situation. In recovery we put down our addiction, only to realize the habits of the mind are still very much alive and well. One of the first insights I had was realizing that I usually felt good in the present based on what had happened or what I thought would happen. The only time I ever felt good for no particular reason was after some exercise. Running with a steady rhythm seemed to do something for me that no amount of thinking ever could. I could not think myself into the present, but I could feel my way into it when I found my pace. After a run, it felt like I had left my "self" behind. I experienced a profound sense of connection with the present moment—the smell of the earth, the sound of the birds, the brush of the wind. There were two worlds, the one my normal mind made and the sacred, natural one I entered after a run. In my second year of recovery, I started running quite a lot.

Reflection

In Zen philosophy, it is said that "we study the self to forget the self." Start to watch the way the self is made. First there is something plain and ordinary, such as a parking space at the end of the street. Then it becomes "your" parking space, and you become a happy you or unhappy you depending on whether or not you get that parking space.

The slow pace of impermanence and unreliability allows us to forget them once in a while. But we so often create a self out of what we are not that once we become aware of this process, it can make our head spin. We are the person with the parking space, we are the person who lost the parking space; we are the person who must correct a wrong by yelling at the driver who took the space; we are the person who regrets yelling; we are the person who still needs a parking space but is now sad because she yelled at a stranger; we are the person who just got a space a lot closer to where we are going; we are the happy person who sees how everything works out in the end; we are the person who showed up on the wrong day.

Mindfulness allows us to watch the mind make up the self as it goes along. Some selves are universal archetypes like the mother, some are main characters, and still others are just passing through. We come to see that the mind-made self is just a placeholder whose purpose is to allow the mind to formulate a response. For the mind to make the "right" decision, it needs a self whose interests it can temporarily serve. Though understandable, it is regrettable because we don't just make up a self. We think this self is who we are, over and over again. To make matters worse, once we have confused this self for who we are, we start to have an emotional life relative to this straw person's fortunes. At this point, compassion comes to the rescue because mindfulness has revealed a dynamic that looks very much like a dog chasing its tail. Compassion offers us the option of giving ourselves a break so that mindfulness can do its job and help us find a way out of a contracted state into a connected one.

Reflection

When we let go, we are letting go of the self and its story, but we do not go anywhere because they are not who we are. Get still, then let go. What are you letting go of?

306.

When the mind moves to create a self with which to measure the world, the body goes along for the ride. Every time this happens, the body pays a price. It contracts into stress patterns as the breath becomes shallow, impairing our ability to rid ourselves of toxins and robbing us of precious energy. While this unfortunate chain of events plays out, our mind is offering our emotional body a version of events that is often quite troubling.

Sitting in mindfulness as this series of consequences plays out is as disturbing as it is confounding. We can't help but make up a self out of the process of making up a self. In this case we are the self that makes up selves while we are supposed to be meditating. We must call upon strength of character to keep coming back to our cushion despite a mind that manages to be both relentless and shameless. If we keep coming back, we start to gain a little inner space. The mind still goes through its loops, but we begin to see that we are not the mind's loops, nor are we the mind's self. Yes, our emotional life is still very much caught up in the mind's stories, and our bodies are still tense, tired, and sore. But we are not as disappointed that the self has made a mess of things again. As we relax, our mind starts to slow down and the power of the mind-made self starts to fade. Each time we relax out of our self, we glimpse a new possibility. Mindfulness starts to be less about what is moving and more about what is not.

Reflection

Twelve-step programs say, "Don't quit before the miracle." The miracle in question is a sober life. The same can be said of meditation, but the miracle in this practice is the insight that you are not your thoughts.

Learning to recognize the three mistakes, formally known as the three forms of suffering, is essentially a lesson in observing something. The Buddha gave us four arenas in which to develop our ability to observe. These arenas constitute the four foundations of mindfulness. Their purpose is for us to be able to readily recognize the nature of our present-moment experience. For training purposes, the Buddha broke down our experience into four domains: body, feelings, thoughts, and mental states. The study of these four domains gives someone practicing mindfulness a sense of what they are trying to accomplish while offering a truly useful form of self-awareness.

Three forms of suffering and four foundations of mindfulness might seem like a lot to keep track of. In practice, it is quite simple. We generally start by resting our attention on the breath while watching as the mind jumps around. Sometimes we are learning how the jumping mind affects us on a physical level (first foundation); sometimes we are learning how the jumping mind affects us on an emotional level (second foundation). In other meditations, we are watching how the moving mind becomes thoughts about what we want and what we do not want (third foundation), and ultimately we learn to watch how the moving mind creates an entire mental state like jealousy or doubt (fourth foundation). We are learning to understand how the habits of our mind affect us on every level. This knowledge helps us to understand how we would think the impermanent is permanent or the unreliable is reliable, or how we would come to believe that what is not the self is the self.

Reflection

A simple form of meditation is to get still and focus on the breath. When the mind moves, note where it moves. Imagine that you are sitting on the bank of a river. Each time the mind moves, imagine it has gotten onto a boat. Name the boat either Planning, Hoping, Doubting, *or* Fearing. *Before long, you will begin to know which boats your mind likes to board.*

308.

"Knowing the body in the body" is a phrase often used when learning the first foundation of mindfulness. When we are sitting, we should know that we are sitting. This seems reasonable. Why would we not want to know that we are sitting when we are sitting? It seems like a bad way to live, not knowing that you are sitting when you are sitting. If you do not know that you are sitting when you are sitting, what could you know? Would you know that anything was true if you did not even know that you were sitting? Wouldn't the fact that you are sitting be the first thing you'd want to know? My teachers certainly felt this way, and they were not shy about telling us about it. To this day, if I am sitting with one of my meditation teachers, the first thing they will tell me is to rest in the felt experience of the body. After I have worked on that for several days, they will let me start to rest in the felt experience of sitting and breathing.

Reflection

Take a seat, upright and relaxed. Then bring steady awareness to the felt experience of the body. For a while, you will choose to experience the still vibrancy of the body. Then if you let go a little more, you will be it.

309.

My first efforts at "knowing the body in the body" were confused at best. The phrase was too simple for my mind to grasp. The idea is that we are no longer trying to know the body as an intellectual construct, such as height, weight, or age. Instead, we are endeavoring, perhaps for the first time, to know the body by bringing our awareness into it. I assumed knowing the body in the body was a mysterious event cloaked in ancient wisdom, or possibly magic. This assuming behavior made the whole thing seem pretty preposterous.

I spent several years trying to do something mysterious, magical, and wise instead of something practical and essential. The first foundation of mindfulness is a simple shift of attention that is sustained so that we can understand something complex. Instead of investing all our energy in the world of our imaginings, we are repurposing that energy to investigate the felt experience of the body. It is a shift—no more, no less. We have been pouring energy into our thoughts; now we will be pouring energy into our connection with the present moment. This repurposing of our energy begins with knowing that we are sitting, walking, tasting, seeing, or smelling.

I did not grasp this simple shift in one blinding moment of insight. I backed into it. There was the warmth of the sun, the smell of the grass, the color of the sky. There was that pain that was my longing to be home but having no idea where that would be. There was my willingness to follow instructions. There were weeks spent sitting in silence with other people. In the end, our relationship with the body is our relationship to the earth beneath our feet and the air in our lungs. The earth welcomed me back the moment I opened my heart to it. Opening the door to that relationship was all that was required.

Reflection

The body is our home as the earth is our home. The first foundation heals this relationship. Feel your desire to heal that relationship. Let yourself feel your desire to be home once again.

310.

The meditation centers where I have trained are set in silent landscapes. The first one I went to was in the middle of the giant forest that is New England. New England's ancient forests do not begrudge us. They seem happy to remind us how old the earth is, how capable it is of holding our pain. It is willing to partner with us, to offer us its stillness, its silence until we can find our own. After a few days of sitting quietly, I would go out into the forest. I had not yet been able to partner with my body, but on those walks, my stillness merged with the presence of the forest. I would stand still to feel how the forest held me, spoke to me, reminded me that I had always been, and would always be, okay.

Reflection

Go outside and listen to the earth.

311.

When I moved to California, I began attending meditation retreats at the Spirit Rock Meditation Center. It rests in the rolling hills of Northern California. When I hike high up in the hills, I can see San Francisco Bay. The forests of New England are cold and wet when they are not hot and wet. The land that holds Spirit Rock is warm and dry. Deer live there, turkeys and foxes too. Memorials to people who have meditated at Spirit Rock and are now missed by loved ones are integrated into the surroundings. Sitting on a bench dedicated to the memory of a young person, I looked into a live oak forest across an open valley. For the first time, I felt how the space held by the valley was as alive as the distant forest or the valley floor. The intimacy with which the valley holds the space, the intimacy with which the space holds the valley, the intimacy with which awareness holds the two things that are one thing became apparent to me as I felt the bench beneath me, the breath within me.

Reflection

Spiritual communities hold the loving-kindness of those who are no longer with us. These ancestors are part of why we succeed. We can do two things to honor them: Receive their love and pass it on.

312.

Mindfulness is the investment of our energy into our connection to the present moment. We stop turning away from the present and start turning toward it. As we spend more time in the present, our mind simultaneously steadies, broadens, and deepens. We start to be able to look closely at aspects of our experience that we did not even know existed before meditation. We become ever closer to our actual potential. This shows up in a dramatic increase in our ability to understand what our teachers are telling us. What may have been a two- or three-year learning curve at the start of our meditation practice often becomes an immediate insight. The teacher explains something, and not only do we understand it, but we begin to embody it skillfully while the talk is still taking place.

We become skillful students, which gives us a passion for life that is not relative to our circumstances; rather, it is relative to the skill with which we are learning to meet them. We come to see that a human is a learner. Meditation has given us ourselves back in the largest sense of the phrase. Mindfulness is both the effort and the experience that make this homecoming possible.

Reflection

Consider what it means for something to be both the effort and the experience. Mindfulness is definitely both. Recovery is as well.

313.

Mindfulness is far more than the ability to reflect on the mind. Mindfulness is the steady cultivation of our connection with the present moment and all of the peace and wonder that connection offers us. But before we can get to the peace and wonder part, we have to learn how to live with our own mind. The addict's plan for that is active addiction. Mindfulness is another plan. While the addict systematically numbs or avoids the mind, the mindfulness practitioner systematically awakens and engages it.

The very first instruction I ever received in mindfulness began with a guided meditation on how to sit while balancing the intention to be calm with the intention to be awake. We learned that we could choose to be awake all day long. Hour after hour—sitting, walking, sitting, eating, sitting, doing one's chores—choosing to be awake. When the Buddha was asked if he was a god or a saint, he said, "I am awake." Three thousand years later, his students are still choosing to be awake. But that is only half of the equation. Being awake is a quality of mind; the other half is a quality of the heart. We practice looking calmly into the world from the moment we wake up to the moment we fall asleep. We learn to be fearless.

Reflection

Sit upright and awake. Then balance that awake quality with the decision to sit calmly. Find the middle. If you are able to do it once, you will be able to do it all day. It will just take a little practice.

314.

Due to the images of the Buddha sitting in calm wisdom, I began meditating with a distorted sense of what I was going to learn. I thought of meditation as an almost bodyless experience in which you transcend everyday concerns. What I found was a much more practical form of education that was almost exaggeratedly embodied. You are learning to sit the way you want to live. When learning a physical skill, you learn in a stable environment, then practice it in increasingly unstable ones. Seated meditation is an extremely stable environment chosen by meditation teachers throughout the ages to teach people how to be in life.

As a mindfulness learning environment, the seated meditation is second to none. Sitting silently, we can look directly at the effect our choices have on us. When we are asked to bring an awake quality to how we are sitting, we can choose to be awake, then we see how that feels. When asked to be calm, we can feel a tranquility settle over us. We can feel what it means to be fearless. Sitting quietly, doing nothing, we can try on ways of being like someone in a clothing store trying on a few different looks for the new school year. How does this fit? How does it feel? Is this something I want to take home with me?

Reflection

Try standing with courage and peace. Then sit with courage and peace. Then choose courage and peace whenever habit would have you choose fear.

315.

One of the challenges we face as we attempt to sit on our cushion in the way we want to stand in our life is that the mind has been dragging our body around for a bunch of decades. This has had a warping effect on the physical body as well as the energy body. I have chosen the word *warp* because I feel that the body without a yoga and meditation practice warps the way untreated wood warps from heat and moisture. Only instead of heat and moisture, the warping is caused by a relentless dynamic of wanting this and fearing that; each time the mind reacts, the body does as well. How often and in what fashion has your mind reacted so far in this lifetime? If you do the math, you will develop a lot of compassion for what your body has been through.

Warped by a lifetime of hope and fear, the body's initial attempts to sit upright for any length of time creates a physical crisis. We hurt here, we ache there; there are endless itches to be scratched. We squirm our way from one end of the meditation to the other. The warping of our physical body means that our energy body is constantly trying to correct itself as it meets one cramped space after the next. All of this correcting is why sitting still is such a whirlwind of unpleasant sensations. Yoga poses can help. They straighten out the physical body, helping the energy body find its optimal flow. Yoga poses also train us to be inwardly aware. A lot of how the energy body corrects itself is with the help of our conscious awareness. Sitting in discomfort, we bring our attention to the stuck point to breathe into it, helping the flow of energy unblock.

Choosing to let go, choosing kindness, choosing courage also helps the flow of energy. Exercise helps. The support of teachers helps, the support of a community helps. Sitting more helps a lot. The decisive factor, however, is our willingness to be calm and awake as the process unfolds, learning how not to react to our habitual reactions. Each time we are still, the warping of our bodies fades a little more. As the spine lengthens, the heart opens.

Reflection

The phrase "The issues are in our tissues" illustrates the link between trauma, addiction, and yoga. Nutrition, exercise, and yoga go a long way in helping an addict work the past out of her body. Now that you are not using, you have a lot more time on your hands. Why not invest in the health and wellness of your body?

316.

As a child, I lived with a very heavy heart. I had been left in an orphanage for two years only to be adopted by a couple who were having a hard time in life. Their unhappiness was overwhelming to me. The world I lived in was obviously mad concerning the color of my skin, even through my young eyes. After a decade or so of my world letting me down, I took over the job myself by drinking and drugging away whatever self-respect I had. Getting sober was a miraculous improvement, but my heart still carried its burden.

I have been taught that we carry the heart's past in our back, right behind the heart. When I came to yoga, my back was so warped with scoliosis that I could not bend backward. With steady effort over a number of years, my back straightened. Eventually I became able to do a full backbend. One of the more intense backbends in yoga is called wheel pose. You lie on your back on the floor, bending your knees to bring your feet under your knees. Then you place your hands, palms down, under your shoulders to lift up into a backbend with only your hands and feet on the floor. This pose radically opens the heart while engaging the muscles behind the heart. For a couple of months, as I became able to move fully into this pose, I would spontaneously cry out a sound that was both sadness and relief. It was such a regular occurrence that I started to do this pose in private. Letting my heart give voice to how it felt to be trapped in a web of suffering was embarrassing in public, but in private it was the best feeling in the world. By the time I was in my mid-30s, backbends had become my favorite poses. To this day, my spine is extremely flexible, offering me a sense of freedom in backbends that I do not experience in any other physical activity.

Reflection

If you are in recovery, you simply have to find a yoga practice that feels good to you.

317.

Of the four foundations of mindfulness, only the first concerns being rooted in the present moment. The remainder address what we discover once we get there. We learn to cultivate our connection to the present moment in the first foundation of mindfulness and continue to cultivate that connection as we begin to study the habits of the mind. This first foundation is the precondition of all the insight, wisdom, and well-being that come as we practice the remaining three foundations.

After a number of years of practice, my experience of this foundation is now central to everything I do. My professional life is dedicated to teaching connection with the present moment as the foundation of all other aspects of spiritual practice. Whether you are living ethically, serving others, gaining insight, or getting sober, you will be doing it in the present. The state of connection to the present moment holds within it a profound well-being in every aspect of our experience. As we enter the moment, the physical body becomes free from tension, the energy body flows freely, the heart finds peace, and the mind rests in non-attached awareness. With practice, we become increasingly able to maintain this state as we go about our everyday lives. Living in this fashion is its own reward. Living in this fashion makes possible the rest of the learning that is mindfulness.

Reflection

We enter recovery because we have to. The alternative is an addict's death. The door we must walk through is marked "Recovery," but what we find on the other side is nothing less than the process of human self-actualization.

318.

Our experience of the present moment is similar to the experience of a diver descending into the depths of the ocean. There is turbulence on the surface; the mind is swept up by every passing wind. Then the diver's attention is absorbed by all the movement just under the surface— the way the fish move, the way the light moves, the way kelp moves. As you dive deeper, you begin to experience pure ocean, ocean without movement. Once we settle into the depths, the fluctuations of the surface no longer disturb us. A world of silence and beauty is revealed. Deeper still lies a darkness from which all else arises. As we approach it, we remember, *I am the darkness.*

Sitting quietly, doing nothing, we watch our thoughts, eventually noticing the awareness that is watching the thoughts. Looking directly at the nature of awareness, we sense the stillness that gives rise to it. Knowing that you are the stillness out of which the moment is born is what it means to be rooted in the present.

Reflection

Sound arises from silence. Movement arises from stillness. Form arises out of emptiness. Rooted in stillness, you close the gap between what could be and what can be.

319.

The insights of the first foundation of mindfulness teach us to recognize the impermanent as impermanent, the unreliable as unreliable, that which is not the self as being truly empty of the self. As we sit quietly, doing nothing, the clouds part and the light of wisdom shines through. Then we get up and the habits of the mind kick in all over again. The knowledge we gain in the first foundation of mindfulness is invaluable, but we still have to deal with the infinity of programmed responses built into our DNA, our ancestral history, and our own difficult life experience. I don't like being cold. I love ice cream. I don't like creepy bugs. I love puppies. I don't like golf. I love surfing. And so it goes, measuring the world by an imaginary self.

The next three foundations of mindfulness use the steady mind we have developed in the first foundation to rid ourselves of greed, hatred, and delusion. It is a patient sort of learning. Much like the naturalist who watches a species in its habitat day after day to understand how the creatures live, we must be careful, respectful, and, above all, motivated by love for what we are observing.

Reflection

We cannot understand that which we do not hold kindly.

320.

As I moved through the skills encompassed in the second, third, and fourth foundations of mindfulness, I was taught to recognize and then accept what was true here and now. There was more to the process, but without the ability to recognize and accept the truth, all other aspects of mindfulness will not serve their purpose. When one is on a Northern California hillside, enduring endless days of sitting in silence, the practice of recognizing and accepting whatever comes up might seem to be a modest pursuit. It is. But the things that matter usually happen modestly, in ordinary settings, in the presence of those we love.

My son loves me with all his heart. When asked who his hero was for a fifth-grade report, he said his father. When asked why, he said because "he is honest with himself." This love from such a beautiful young person is precious to me beyond words. I earn it one day at a time under his watchful eye by being willing to know what is true here and now, then living up to it. I worked with children for years before my son was born. From them I learned that an honest adult is all children are asking for. Sitting quietly, learning mindfulness, we are practicing a form of beauty that will eventually find its home between two hearts.

Reflection

We bridge the distance between us by being honest and kind. This is why meetings work. This is how mindfulness works. This is what a relationship looks like in recovery, whether it is with ourselves, our loved ones, our boss at work, or the person behind the counter at the gas station.

Chapter Eight

Concentration

Bill Wilson offered his community an important support as it gathered to address the problem of addiction. He taught that a 12-step program should have a "singleness of purpose." People come to a 12-step program to work on their addiction. A concentrated focus allows for excellence in addressing the problem. The success a 12-step member experiences when putting down a substance or stopping negative behavior provides a steady foundation on which to stand while addressing the many other challenges on the path of recovery. In this chapter, we will discuss how a singleness of purpose can support an infinity of choices.

321.

In her seminal work on the chakras, *Creating on Purpose*, Anodea Judith wrote that to create anything, we must accept limitation. From an infinite number of options, we must choose one and pursue it. Before we choose, we entertain the pleasure of having many options. To follow the one path, we must let go of that pleasure. In order to create, we must be willing to feel the pain of limitation. Learning to sit with a necessary discomfort is not part of the addict's playbook, so when we come into recovery, we have to learn it. Going to meetings helps a lot. We share time, follow rules, attempt temperate speech, and generally try to be law-abiding so that we can create a connection to a community that will help us survive. We discover the role of discipline in creating a life worth living.

The first disciplines we learn in a 12-step program are parallel to the external disciplines in yoga because they concern what is done outside the body as opposed to what happens inside. We are taught to sit up front, raise our hands, and plan our day around a meeting. We are taught to have "sober feet" even when our heads could not be exactly called sober. We learn it is enough to have sober feet that walk away from experiences that challenge our recovery and into experiences that support our recovery. We are taught how to live out of one life into another.

Reflection

What does it mean to you to plan your day around your recovery? My friend Tommy Rosen says, "If you don't have a plan to stay sober, you have a plan." When he says that to a group of addicts, it always get a laugh of surprised recognition because Tommy is bringing to light the fact that the addict has always had a plan. Recovery means that she has to have a new plan or live out the old one.

322.

When I got sober, I had been around discipline for much of my life. I went to old, prestigious schools that were steeped in passion for devoted study. I played on good sports teams with inspired peers coached by present, informed coaches. From these experiences, I plunged into a number of years in the U.S. Army infantry. It can rightly be said that I had been exposed to as much discipline as is humanly possible in the first couple of decades of my life, though sadly very little of it got through the cloud of my addiction.

The military did the best job of getting through to me, possibly because I would have to go out into the woods for months at a time, so I was not drinking while I was trying to learn. The types of discipline I learned from the military only transferred to my personal life after I had been in recovery for a while. For example, I learned a tremendous amount of discipline by using a map and a compass. Most of it amounted to recognizing that I often didn't check my math and that I'd have to make an effort to do so. This discipline has transferred nicely when I have had to get somewhere or learn something new. Double-checking what you think you know is a good habit. I learned many organizational disciplines from the military, but I was tone-deaf to personal disciplines the way addicts are when they are using. It was not until I began sitting in meetings listening to people talk about their lives that it occurred to me that you could have a plan for your day that encompassed both what you would do and how you would do it.

Reflection

Name a discipline you learned before coming into recovery. Name the discipline you are learning today.

At first, it would have been hard to tell whether I was motivated, disciplined, or just very scared. I adhered to my program of recovery, or my sober disciplines, like a drowning man holding on to a life preserver. I was not so much embracing a set of disciplines to make my life work as I was doing whatever I could to stay alive.

After my first year of sobriety, things started to calm down, which provided me with an opportunity to try this or that and see how things felt. I tried going door-to-door to raise money for the environment and hated it. I waited tables and loved it. I went to meetings every day and felt inspired. I would skip a meeting and go slowly mad. I tried romance and it was a mess. I tried friendship and it was deeply rewarding. A fan of feeling good, I started to have a passion for behaviors that led to positive outcomes. Some of these were one-offs, like watching a particular movie. Others were more regular occurrences, like getting enough sleep or going to certain meetings. I had some time on my hands, so it was not long before I had tried a number of behaviors. I would continue the ones that seemed to work out and abandon the ones that did not. Before long, it felt like I had a life, which meant that I had a plan for a sober day that was part of my plan for a sober week. Twenty-seven years later, it has not yet been necessary to have a plan for a sober month. My plan meant that I had to make certain sacrifices. If I wanted to make a particular meeting, I could not sleep in. If I wanted to take an opportunity at work, I had to adjust my meeting schedule. I began learning how to accept limitation in order to create a sober day.

Reflection

Write down your ideal sober day.

324.

To get sober, I had to make recovery from addiction my number-one priority. Everything else in my life had to support this priority. My living situation, my employment, my friendships, my every waking hour of every day was directly accountable to this main priority in my life. This is singleness of purpose. Twelve-step programs help us approach life by breaking it down into simple slogans. We are to put "first things first" then "live one day at a time." If other people's choices are troublesome, we are to mind our own business, not get drawn into drama, learning over time to "live and let live." These three slogans support us in directing our energy toward the single purpose of recovery.

As a newcomer, I found myself amid a crew of other newcomers who expressed different levels of satisfaction with this purpose. Some felt they did not really need to work that hard. Some felt they could not work that hard. Still others felt that the people in the meetings were lame, so following their example was pointless. I belonged to another part of the new crowd, those who had decided to follow the instructions. What we found was that you can't really know the value of something until you experience it firsthand. Applying the slogans to the challenges of everyday life worked out pretty much perfectly every time. We also discovered two things that can be experienced only after a discipline has been applied over some time: There are behaviors that give back more energy than you put into them, and each time you choose them, it makes it easier to choose them the next time.

Reflection

If you had to live by only two slogans, what would they be?

325.

The Buddha dedicated much of his teachings to the concept of concentration. He described a concentrated mind as collected and unified. To reach that state, we collect our mental energy and bring it to bear on a single purpose. In my work, I use a number of terms to convey the power of a concentrated mind with regard to the challenges of everyday life. I encourage people to give their undivided attention to the process of learning, to be of one mind, to speak with one voice when they work together.

Imagine what it means for us to be collected, unified, of one mind, one heart, one purpose—not in the service of some peak experience but in the service of our daily responsibilities. Imagine the satisfaction that comes when we are able to bring the sacred power of an unconflicted mind to bear on the ordinary acts of loving-kindness that make up our daily existence in recovery. This is a possibility that is worthy of investigation.

Reflection

To act with one mind, to be whole-hearted. Is there a difference?

326.

Teaching yoga gave me my first experiences of the power of an undivided mind. At first, there was the sense of flow that one would expect, the days when everything came together. Then I started being able to adjust to the unexpected, turning whatever came up in class into the best possible outcome. Later I learned how a steady mind makes room for inspiration. We quiet the individual mind to be able to listen to the universal one. Eventually, I started running teacher trainings that often entailed teaching for 10 hours at a time instead of 1 or 2. In this setting, I discovered that a concentrated mind did not really tire. One day when I was quite sick, I asked someone to drive me to a workshop because I knew that once I got into the room, I would be able to access the power of a collected mind. Although I could not have driven a car, I was able to lead that workshop with the same ease as any other I had ever led.

I believe I am approaching the end of the first stage of my journey as a teacher, the stage in which we find our calling. I believe I am starting to teach what I was born to teach because I have learned how to work with my own mind. I am familiar with the subtle effort that keeps our attention on the present for hours at a time. I am able to receive the messages from the quantum field that encompasses the energy bodies of all the people in the room. But most of all, I am familiar with how a quiet mind invites the universal mind, how to ask the question, how to listen for the answer. This partnership with the universal mind comes to us for two reasons. The first is that we work at it. We take the time to bring our attention back to the present moment after moment, day after day, year after year. The second reason is the more important one. We learn to act with one mind because it is what is needed to serve others. Our greatest asset as we develop an unconflicted mind is our desire to be of service. Rooted in that desire, we will find an effort that outlasts our challenges.

Reflection

We do our best when we know that our efforts can benefit others. We recognize this even in early recovery, when we remember that any good we will do with the rest of our lives hinges on what we do now. Remember that you are in recovery not simply for yourself but for everyone you will help in the years to come.

327.

The speed with which I adapted my mind to the challenges of teaching yoga was in no way matched by the speed with which I adapted my mind to the challenges of everyday life. I would teach for days on end in an ever-increasing state of grace, then come home to the patterns, losses, and traumas that had warped my life. For a while, I hoped that it would be enough for me to be great at something. Being great at something seemed easier to accomplish than being okay in my own skin. Then my daughter was born, and my off-line existence became the only game in town. I had been living to work, but now I would have to learn how to work to live.

The truth was that I was not really all that good at being off-stage. With the support of a challenge and people to serve, I could let go of the fact that I had not really made peace with anything. I had not made peace with my childhood. I had not made peace with my addiction. I had not made peace with the deaths of those closest to me or with my own survival. When I was not teaching, the many conflicts in my heart dominated my inner life. My mind was in a permanent state of distraction over the unresolved pain of my life. Ice cream helped, as well as lots of exercise, movies, nature, and a wonderful partner. All of these made me feel less alone, less sad, less conflicted, but if you looked closely, you would see a child with a broken heart. This is not what I wanted my daughter to see when she looked at her father. I wanted my daughter to see that I could live with one mind, one heart, one purpose. I believed that I could because I believed that others had. Now it was my time to find out how.

Reflection

As active addicts, we lived to use. In recovery, we often find ourselves living to work. Ultimately, though, recovery is about learning to work to live. How is that going for you?

328.

I am writing these words on a Veterans Day weekend. Social media is filled with images of people in uniform who have grown old. In their faces you can see the brilliance of youth. If we look closely into their eyes, the light of the spirit is there for all to see. So is the karma that creates the path on which we walk through life. There is the light, and then there are circumstances the light finds itself in. A human life is a dance between the light of the spirit and the burden of karma.

Consider how one child is born into abject poverty while another is born into wealth or how one struggles with poor health while another enjoys good health. At the level of spirit, each child is the same. The light is the same in each pair of eyes. The light is the same, but the circumstances are not.

Reflection

We learn to bloom where we are planted. It feels both humbling and empowering to be willing to work with what you have, to choose faith instead of fear, to trust that the great opportunity is where you are, and to believe that the light within you has chosen this time, this place.

I attended my first meditation retreats in response to becoming a father. My circumstances had changed dramatically. My behavior was going to impact someone in a way that I had never contemplated before. In addition to this new pressure was the fact that my parents had made it clear to me that who one is as a parent is more important than what one says. I was now someone who was teaching another person about the world with what I held in my heart. Due to the intensity of the reasons that brought me to meditation retreats, I had not given much thought to what I was going to learn.

Sitting through my first difficult days, I was taught to bring my mind to the present, to do it again and again. I was instructed to do that one simple behavior all day long, even when I was going to sleep. Later I would learn that this is the first stage of concentration. The second stage is learning to rest in the connection to the present you make in the first stage. The first two stages are likened to striking a bell, then listening to the reverberations. In the midst of an adult life passing through a transformative flexion point, I was asked to notice the breath as it came in and then as it came out all day long. As this practice started to set in, I was instructed to savor my experience of being alive. Instead of grabbing on to my experience, I was told to rest in it—to rest in the experience of the in breath, to rest in the experience of the out breath. Walking on creaky floors in thick, big winter socks, I began to rest in a felt experience—a sound, a taste, a smell, the colors of a winter sunset. The third stage is called rapture. It is likened to the feeling someone has in the desert when glimpsing an oasis on the horizon.

Reflection

If we bring our attention into the present moment with enough regularity, it will start feeling like water in the desert.

330.

Each of the first three stages of concentration have had their own moment in my life. For a while, I just toughed it out by bringing my attention back to the breath day after day. I might have been wearing loose, comfortable clothing, drinking tea in nubby socks, but I was in the battle of my life. My mind wanted to go in one direction, but my heart refused. The enjoyment that came from this phase was mostly from knowing that I was in the right place doing the right thing. Having gone to rehab and 12-step meetings, I knew what a blessing it was to be in the right place at the right time.

The second and third stages of concentration happened one right after the other. I started to hear people saying things like "relax into the present" and "soften, ease, and allow." Exhausted from my battle, I tried letting things be easy. The phrase "rest in the felt experience of the body" was a game changer. There is a profound shift when we stop clinging to our experience in favor of resting in it. This allowed me to get into the habit of receiving the fullness of an experience. I would put down my spoon, sit back, breathe, to receive what this spoonful of soup actually tasted like. I learned that receiving included how it felt to be receiving the taste of soup. I saw that beneath the places where my heart had been broken, I had a heart that could still be delighted by the taste of soup. Resting in a heart that could still be delighted by life, I understood why the third stage of concentration was called rapture.

Reflection

We think we are a noun, but we are a verb; we are a process. This is certainly true when it comes to being brokenhearted. The heart is a process.

331.

The experience of concentration unfolds in stages. I learned to choose connection through one of the five senses, then rest in that connection. These skills encompass the first two stages of concentration. While resting in connection with the present moment, a new possibility can be glimpsed. Life can regain its magic, its mystery, its childlike wonder. This glimpsing is felt rapturously, hence the name of the third stage of concentration. In the fourth stage, that which was glimpsed becomes a reality. This stage is called happiness.

I feel it is important to note that as a person in recovery, you have just been told that happiness happens when we start to rest in reality. One of the most luminous minds in human history has laid out a path for us to follow to happiness. But it is entirely up to us. We do not need anything we do not already have. We simply need to turn our attention toward the present moment. We need to learn to rest in the present as opposed to trying to grab at it. Wisdom knows the destination, intention knows the direction, wise effort moves us there.

Reflection

In 12-step programs, recovery is an "inside job." In yoga, it is said that "the pose is what you are doing; yoga is how you are being in the pose." In meditation, we learn to be in the body and the breath the way we want to be in life.

332.

I did not know that I was experiencing rapture or even what I was experiencing. One minute I was practicing walking meditation, the next I was home. Home under the summer stars with my pulse matching the pulse of the night around me. These episodes of awe started to happen more often after that, when I would step entirely out of time into a vibrant eternal moment. After they passed I would try to regain them, to *get* something that I could only *be*. Once I let go of trying, the moments would come back. The Yoga Sutras say that we are not seeing things as they are. Rapture is the moment when we begin to see. In Zen this is called satori, the moment of clarity in which we gain insight into the truth of our existence. For me these moments created a space in my broken heart that had not been there before. *Hope* is too small a term for what this space let in.

Coming home, I had to adjust to a world lost in the belief that getting the next desired thing was as good as it gets. I had to learn to walk a fine line—bills had to be paid, soccer games had to be attended, the duties of life had to be fulfilled. However, why I went about those duties changed. It is said that the Buddha conquered death and achieved the deathless state. I do not know anything about that, but by the time I was in my early 40s, I could no longer fear death. I could only fear not having lived. To become truly still is to make a friend of nonexistence. While the world around me clung to things, I had found the freedom of the no-thing. No longer able to live in fear, I had to learn what it meant to live for love.

Reflection

I heard in 12-step meetings that religion is for those who fear hell, while spirituality is for those who have already been there. Finding stillness is a major milestone on the way back from hell.

333.

Each of the first four stages of concentration was challenging for me because of my penchant for wanting the impermanent to be permanent, wanting the unreliable to be reliable, and making a self out of that which was not the self. I would have a moment or two of clarity, resting in the bliss of being, feeling the wonder of rapture. Then I would jump ahead, wanting to be the self that felt that way all the time, after which I would be upset that what I wanted was impermanent and unreliable.

My mind was in constant flux, but what made matters worse was the way I was in a constant state of reaction to the fluctuations of my mind. I had to abandon the notion of permanent bliss and find a little patience with myself. It turned out that changing the way my mind processed reality was a big deal. If I wanted success, I would have to be my own coach, my own best friend, my own cheering section. The first steps I took in that direction were simple yet effective. I learned to:

A. Redefine success as showing up and participating wholeheartedly. My goal was to participate with a good attitude. If I did that, I was winning.

B. Acknowledge the skillful mental states I experienced, however briefly, as successes in their own right. Otherwise, I would not be able to learn from them.

Reflection

By developing the skill of concentration, one discovers the capacity for non-attached participation.

334.

In the early stages of practicing concentration, we experience mind states the way the shadows of clouds pass over a field. Their existence is a lesson in impermanence. Working with the mind flickering from clarity to confusion and from contraction to connection requires us to be steadfast and patient. For many of us, wise effort is our first breakthrough. We find we can "hold on loosely," keeping the attention fairly steady while letting go of the expectation that our experience should be this way or that way. Mindfulness comes next as we develop a sensitivity to the disruption of a mind that has left the present. We become steady in our desire to abide in the present.

Concentration stands on the shoulders of wise effort and mindfulness, affording us a view into the nature of the moment that we could not have without them. Wise effort has made us steady. Mindfulness has made us present. Concentration asks, "Is there wisdom here? In this choice, this action, this path?" As these three abilities develop, we find ourselves able to know the answer to this simple question. Even as the mind flashes from one state to another, chaotically unfolding like the patterns of raindrops in a puddle, we find ourselves able to know if the path we are on is leading to suffering or well-being.

Reflection

The question we were born to ask is "Is there wisdom here?" Living into the answer, we find the change we were born to be in the world.

335.

As we learn to abide in the present moment, we discover an authentic path to happiness. At first, it was hard for me to trust that my life could be that simple or good. When I began going to 12-step meetings, it was clear that I was among people who had found something worthwhile. This same feeling was even more noticeable as I took my place among the Yogis. While practicing yoga in the spectacular setting of the Berkshire Mountains, my heart would leap for joy as my eyes filled with tears of gratitude.

Even so, taking my seat with 100 other meditators for nine days in silence felt like taking the SATs. In 12-step meetings it was obvious that I belonged; on the yoga mat my athletic training gave me a lot of confidence. But working with my mind in silence was another thing entirely.

While yoga and 12-step practice played to my strengths, meditation seemed to require abilities that I had very little experience with. I came from a volatile, unstable lot who let their passions sweep them into rage, melancholy, and addiction. There was nothing I could point to that led me to believe I would be able to train my mind. The only thing I had going for me was that I was not much of a quitter. Given half a chance, I will keep coming back. This sort of courage does not guarantee excellence, but it will always lead to progress. Happiness has come to me in fits and starts.

I lost the ability to worry, then I found the ability to forgive. As my brain healed from trauma and addiction, my teachers started making sense. The transition from retreat to home became less of a challenge as my practice became my way of life. Perhaps the last stage has been the gathering of my energy into the present. These days if I am not enjoying each step of a process, I slow down until I am, even when I am leaving the car to get the groceries out of the back or taking trips back and forth. These are the moments to enjoy the sun on my face, the grace of the life I am living now, the vibrant timelessness inherent in any experience. In happiness, concentration deepens.

Reflection

The happiness of recovery happens like leaves falling from a tree. Soundless, seemingly random, a process is in motion that will bring you love, joy, and meaning. Name a couple of the leaves that have fallen recently for you.

336.

As the Buddha studied the nature of his experience, he discovered the relationship between connection, happiness, and concentration. Concentration is an expression of a tremendous amount of focused energy. We have to collect our energy into the present if we want to sustain our attention on the present in a way that will facilitate learning, growth, or insight. Wise effort and mindfulness deliver a steady connection with the present moment, which liberates us from the suffering of the distracted mind. Buoyed by the magnificence of the present moment, we move from rapture to happiness, a true sort of happiness that is derived from the bliss of being.

You see this in action at 12-step meetings, which are buoyed by the joy of recovery humming in the room from people who have spent the past decade or so at a spiritual nadir only to find themselves able to focus, learn, empathize, and participate in a complex social setting with skill. Listening to our peers share their experiences, strength, and hope, we find that we have the heart for any challenge.

Reflection

The quality of your experience is related to the quality of your attention. My teachers encourage me to pay exquisite attention to what I am doing while I walk, sit, eat, or attend to a chore. This leads to happiness in everyday life. Try it.

337.

Over the years, I have appreciated certain adages long before I understood their full meaning. One of them has been "We think that if we succeed, we will be happy, but it is only after we learn to be happy that we will succeed." I have always loved the paradoxical nature of this saying, how it draws our attention to happiness as existing separately from a particular outcome or circumstance. I also love how it points to happiness as something that you can learn. One may not have mastered it yet, but it's never too late to start learning how to be happy.

Progress in meditation has deepened my understanding of the relationship between happiness and success. When you begin to sit regularly, you will notice an elevation in your mood. Research has shown that this is in part due to actual brain growth that you experience from regular meditation. I have found that this elevation of my mood is directly related to the amount of time I spend with my attention on the present instead of the past, the future, or a delusion. As the amount of time I spend in the present increases, the amount of energy I lose absorbed in pointless mental activity decreases. The elevation of my mood has matured into a general gladness to be alive. As this gladness has taken hold, I no longer seek success because I no longer seek anything. The energy of seeking has been rechanneled into the desire to serve a world whose pain no longer has the capacity to break my heart. At this point, I have collected and unified my energy. The distinctions between concepts like recovery, happiness, or success have fallen away as the purity of my heart's intention steps out into the light.

Reflection

A spiritual practice like 12-step or yoga contains the tools we need to create happiness in our lives. Which tools are you applying to create happiness in your life?

338.

It has been an enormous privilege to spend time with three of the great spiritual traditions, traditions that come from humanity's pain and express humanity's genius. Within the worlds they have created, I have found my recovery and my purpose. Bill Wilson spoke of the need for a singleness of purpose. This has been true for me. I have needed to put first things first. I have needed a straightforward, simple life in which to get sober. This singleness of purpose has led to a life of profound happiness.

The Buddha charted a course to freedom that has been followed by countless individuals over thousands of years. In it, he explains how we can turn toward the present moment with such consistency that our heart will eventually find liberation. This has been true for me. Sitting in stillness, I became stillness. Looking directly at awareness, I became awareness. Stepping into the present, I stepped out of the prison of my mind. I experienced this freedom with an elation that has matured into happiness containing a profound sense of purpose. Walking in the shadow of my teacher's teachers, I have found the great circle.

Reflection

One of the joys of 12-step recovery is that it is not aligned with any particular spiritual tradition. Rather, it is aligned with health in any form it takes. This allows us to see the beauty each tradition holds, becoming a living crossroads of spiritual practice. Treasure your role in all of this. You are the place where everything connects.

339.

The question of active addiction is: "Is there relief here?" The question of recovery is: "Is there wisdom here?" In active addiction, the best we can hope for is a night of relief. Our lives are reduced to a search for a temporary reprieve from a life in search of a temporary reprieve. It is a path with zero return on the investment we make in it. As the years go by, this has drastic consequences, not the least of which is that the life skills we accumulate living this way result only in the ability to get the next fix. It is no wonder that people entering recovery benefit from gatherings dedicated to discussing sober life skills.

It is miraculous that someone who has lived this way has the will to live at all. It is a further miracle that this person will readily develop an interest in the cultivation of wisdom. But we do. Sitting in church basements, we discover a question resting in a forgotten corner of our soul. "Is there wisdom here?" starts out as just a whisper in the din of our self-reproach. As the months in recovery accumulate, the whisper becomes a chorus in the background as we sit in meetings or work with a sponsor, therapist, yoga teacher, or friend. Listening to this whisper becomes the point of much of what we do. One day we find ourselves being asked to sit silently to watch the breath come in and then go out. Listening inwardly is the point; if we stop listening, even for a moment, we are to stop and begin again. In time, we discover that we are a verb, not a noun. We are a process that is learning to listen for the sound of wisdom.

Reflection

The next time you are in the presence of spiritual teachings, ask yourself, "Is there wisdom here?" Then notice that you will know whether there is or not.

340.

It's hard to say when I began developing concentration in my life. At 14, I spent the first of many summers running to the gym three times a week, getting ready for football that fall. The jogs were in the summer heat; the workouts were repetitive. In order to be consistent, I had to turn the tedious into something special. I planned ahead, being as creative as I could be with the design of my workouts. By making it fun, I found that the time went quickly. I began looking forward to the next workout. Later, during long, intense military training, I learned to let go of the future or the desire for anything in particular—the less mental activity, the better. Before long I could fall asleep on the way to a night parachute jump.

Once I got to meetings, I found that the rigors of difficult training, whether for a sport or in the military, had taught me some useful mental disciplines. I had learned how to make a repetitive process fun. I had learned to appreciate the small gains one makes in the midst of a larger commitment. I had learned to reduce an experience to its component parts, then tackle each one in turn. I had learned to learn. Sitting in my first meetings, I was not afraid of big challenges because I knew that they could be broken down into a series of smaller ones. Once you broke something down, it was easy to see how each small step mattered. Living this way, I had learned to see the opportunity in the ordinary moment. Recovery was simply another set of ordinary moments to be met with all I had.

Reflection

How has life prepared you for the work of recovery?

341.

My coaches would break a complex concept like a football game or a wrestling match down to its component parts. From an educational standpoint, any other method was a nonstarter. Really, you can teach someone only one thing at a time. Having established a singleness of purpose, my coaches would then further break down a component part of the sport, such as a single-leg takedown or an off-tackle run, into specific physical skills that could be drilled repeatedly.

This continual refinement of the educational process toward a single action to be practiced was not a result of deep Yogic practices. My coaches were practical men who hoped to support young people as they worked toward their goals. They had learned from their own experience how hard it is to learn something new. They had learned from thousands of hours working with athletes that if someone was going to understand something, it would require the right setting and the right mind-set.

The coach's job was to provide a focused setting. The athlete's job was to bring the right mind-set. This mind-set has two qualities. The first is that it is undivided. Athletes have to learn to let go of everything else in their lives in order to give the skill they are learning their full attention. The second quality of the right mind-set is that it involves being utterly absorbed. The sports world has coined the phrase "being in the zone" to describe this quality of an athlete's performance. For us to gain the insight for a new understanding to take hold, the mind must be intimately connected to what is true here, now. By practicing the same routines over and over again, an athlete has the opportunity to refine what she is doing *and* how she is being. Over time she learns to connect the experience of how she is being with the results she is seeing.

Reflection

Make a list of the five life skills you need to practice to support your recovery. Then identify the three most important skills on that list. Then select the most important one of the three. Give this skill your undivided attention during set moments of your day, such as at a meeting or driving to work. Then connect deeply to the felt experience of living from this skill.

Because a sport amounts to an intense learning process, athletes who succeed have learned to learn. This means that they have developed many positive qualities. They have the ability to work with others. They have self-honesty. They have resiliency in the face of setbacks. All of them possess an almost uncanny ability to concentrate.

Concentration is a hallmark of the greats. It becomes a habit of their minds. Being in a fairly deep state of concentration has allowed them to listen excellently to the subtle aspects of whatever they are being taught. In action they combine inspired creativity and unflappable equanimity with a perfect economy of effort. When the mind is in concentration, nothing is wasted. Opportunity is observed and acted upon, action is taken without an ounce of extra effort, the chaotic nature of life is experienced as a series of options leading to the intended outcome. When I observe the excellence these individuals are able to attain, I am not deterred by the obvious fact that they possess special abilities. The concentration they have developed is not due to their unique abilities; rather, it is a result of their unique circumstances. These are individuals who have chosen to be in a situation in which learning is the only way forward.

Reflection

Consider the relationship between learning and recovery. Then consider the relationship between learning and the ability to pay attention. What opportunities do you have to practice paying attention?

343.

The military uses many of the same educational strategies as sports but with a slightly different emphasis. While athletic coaches stress team spirit, the assumed primary motive in sports is individual success. An athlete trains to experience personal success. Her sense of kinship with her team helps her overcome the challenges in her path, but her path leads toward personal excellence. The military cannot rely on this ultimate goal. For many in military training, the outcome may be positive for the team but lethal for the individual. Accordingly, the military relies on your investment in those around you as your primary motive for giving your training a full effort. You focus on the matter at hand because other people's lives are at stake. When you know others will benefit from your actions, you pay attention just as well as you do when the goal is your own success—if not better.

In the sports world, the quintessential image is of an individual moving effortlessly in the zone, achieving personal goals in a fashion that exceeds all ordinary expectations. In the military, you will more often see a group of people calmly "sticking to their guns," dying in anonymity so that others may live. There is something entirely compelling about a human being overcoming adversity, and it is hard to say which image stirs my heart more. In sports, the definition of success is the realization of human potential, while in the military success is the preservation of it.

Reflection

We concentrate when we are properly motivated. This proper motivation can be found in the effort to realize your own potential or to preserve that potential in others. What is motivating you today?

344.

During my first year of recovery, my focus was primarily on my own survival. This often boiled down to getting my next chip. Within the larger 12-step community, there are regional differences. In my region, a person in the first year would get a chip to represent a length of sobriety. These chips were handed out for one month, then three, six, nine months, and finally one year. After that, it was a medallion for each year of sobriety. During my first 10 years of recovery, getting a medallion was the biggest thing that would happen to me all year.

After I received my one-year medallion, I spent a month or two adjusting to the fact that I might actually live. Small indicators started showing up. I had to replace a pair of sneakers I had bought in early sobriety. I realized they were the first item of clothing I had worn sober from start to finish. The sneakers were quickly followed by a series of other items, friendships, and activities that belonged solely to my sober life. As my second sober summer turned into my second sober fall, I began noticing another change. Newcomers began showing up at meetings—this one had one month, this one had three. I came to know them. I knew their stories; I knew when they would get six months. I looked forward to watching them succeed. I began to see myself as a part of these newcomers' support system. Their presence inspired me to model healthy participation in the process of the meeting. By my second sober winter, I was no longer solely focused on my own success. Meetings were now a place where joy filled my heart when others succeeded.

Reflection

A healthy spiritual community affords us a chance to have our success celebrated and to celebrate the success of others. This joyful connection is one of the things I was looking for in my active addiction but did not find until I was in active recovery. I believe it is a hallmark of active recovery.

345.

My coaches taught me to break a movement down into a set of skills. This would enable me to concentrate on a specific learning until it was mastered. My military trainers taught me to draw strength from my sense of accountability to the others who were relying on me. Focused on a specific skill, motivated by a desire to serve, I experienced a highly effective mind-body state.

Replicating this level of participation in recovery took a while. My first few years were dedicated to figuring out who I was. I worked jobs that did not require me to think or feel very much. When I was ready to be of service, my motivation was no longer to achieve personal success or to protect my country. I was now part of something that transcended the boundaries of the world I knew before recovery. Describing a friend, Bill Wilson had written 70 years before that "his roots grasped new soil." When I walked back into a classroom to learn how to help other addicts, I knew what he was talking about. It is one of the largest gifts of recovery to have our roots in the soil of a truly profound purpose. I would break down whatever I was taught into individual skills to be mastered. I would never forget those who were counting on me. Still newly sober, I found that I could use these disciplines in the service of a purpose that seemed to be the very purpose of humanity.

Reflection

We are beginning to create a checklist of factors that support concentration.
A) Do one thing at a time.
B) Do it for love.

346.

At meetings during my first few years of sobriety, I could not take on anything more challenging than making the coffee because of the extent of my post-traumatic stress. I was a mess the day I got sober, but the death of my sister from an overdose six months later sent me over the edge. I stayed sober through her funeral and the hard months that followed, but I was not actually present for anything other than what was going on in the meetings. At meetings, the extreme loss I felt was met with empathy. Everywhere else, it was met with fear or incredulity. When I was alone, the despondency I experienced felt permanent. The skills I had learned from sports and the military were largely absorbed by the effort it took me to get out of bed in the morning.

Stepping onto a yoga mat offered me another way to prepare myself for the challenges of everyday life. Sports and military training focused on external behavior. The goals in both of these disciplines are accomplished in the physical world. Yoga was my first life training that focused entirely on my inner life, my experience of being alive. The goal was not a pose; it was my experience of the pose. When I first stepped onto my mat, I had given up on the experience of being alive. Happiness was for people who had not been woken up and brought to see their dead sister, her lips blue from asphyxiation. I was planning on gratitude for my recovery to get me through the days of living I had left. During one of my first few classes, a teacher asked me to feel into my shoulder to see if there was any tension present. Then he said I should breathe into it to release the tension. I did as I was told. The tension lessened a little, but my life changed entirely. Resting on my back in a room full of people, I began to learn how to take care of myself. I had learned how to catch a pass; I had learned how to read a map. Now I was being taught to move toward my pain with compassion.

Reflection

In meetings, I was taught to hold my pain with compassion from the neck up. This got me sober. On my mat, I learned how to do it with the rest of my body. This got me present.

347.

By holding a yoga posture, I learned to follow extremely subtle guidance. My teacher told me to be strong here, be relaxed there, feel this, let go of that. As profoundly practical as this type of training was, it has taken me decades to understand it. Walking into my first few classes, my attention was drawn to the appearance of things. My mind quickly built a story out of how things hit my senses. Yoga smelled like this, looked like this, was supposed to be this way. The narrative I created in the early years on my mat nearly obscured the healing that was taking place. Even so, a friendship was slowly forming between my heart and life itself.

Quiet moments were occurring when I felt the beauty of life. I did not understand what they meant. I felt they were something I had to earn and would often despair over being good enough to get these moments on a permanent basis. Despite my misunderstanding, these glimpses kept me coming back to my mat. In time I understood where these moments were taking place. *The beauty of life happens here.* I also began to understand when they happen. *The beauty of life happens now.* The moment came when I understood the story of Adam and Eve being cast out of the garden as a story only a human would tell another human out of pain and confusion. I knew long before I could speak the truth of it that we have never left the garden. At this point, when my teachers asked me to feel this or that, I understood why they would ask such a thing. The day came that I could hear what my teachers felt in their hearts: "See, the garden is here, and it is here as well. Feel the garden in your breath, feel the garden beneath your feet, feel how you are the garden. It is time to remember who you are."

Reflection

It is time to remember who we are.

In a 12-step program, you slowly reassemble your life. It begins with the detoxification process. After a few weeks the mind-body begins to heal. At a month into sobriety, I had a functional form of mental clarity. Learning began in earnest. With a clear head, I could apply the wisdom I was hearing in meetings to the everyday decisions that would add up to my early recovery. I built my life around recovery; my day around a meeting; my character around honesty, open-mindedness, and willingness. My mind-body healed very quickly, but at times it felt as if my heart would never heal.

On a yoga mat, you slowly reassemble your heart. It begins with a relearning process of standing, sitting, inhaling, exhaling, developing a steady gaze. With a strong body and a steady gaze, I could eventually apply the wisdom of my teachers to the subtle shifts that would add up to ending my war with life. I built my life around connection, my day around the practice of connection, my heart around the experience of connection. The healing of my heart has been a very slow process. For this I am grateful because I have been able to feel all of it.

Reflection

Recovery *is a verb, not a noun. A practice sets things in motion. What are you setting in motion today?*

349.

As my heart healed, it became clear to me that I had habits of the mind that were not in support of the life I was creating for my family or myself. In particular, thinking or acting from anger felt aberrant. I understood how sorrow or disappointment came with the territory of a human life. I could understand desire, attachment, and jealousy, but there was a quality to my anger that did not feel justified. The narrative of the anger I inherited from my angry family tree was "I am the judge; I decide what should be or should not be. As the judge, I say, *'This should not be!'*" This narrative felt at odds with my spiritual beliefs concerning "turning my will and my life over to the care of God as I understand God." Moving into this mind state felt like a vehement rejection of my heart's desire for connection.

By taking my seat at my first meditation retreat, I had signed on to work on a lot more than my anger, but I was going to have to develop a healthy relationship with it first. Yoga had taught me how to feel. This turned out to be excellent preparation for meditation. Sitting quietly, doing nothing, I was visited by all of the felt states that move through me during an ordinary day. I was bored, I was intrigued, I was planning, I was hopeful, I was prideful, and I was pissed off.

Feeling into anger as a mind state, I recognized the imperious child-king quality that I had already recognized on my mat. "I want what I want now!" Beneath the child king was the aggrieved party. Beneath the aggrieved party was a person who was trying to make things right. Beneath the person who was trying to make things right was the person who was in pain and did not know what to do. My sister's last words were "I don't know what to do." Sitting quietly, feeling into the stillness of a cool morning, I felt what it was like to be my sister, I felt what it was like to be my parents, I felt what it was like to be the firemen in Birmingham who had turned their hoses on schoolchildren, I felt what it was like to be the parents of those children. I have not escaped my anger, but I have become willing to learn what it can teach me.

Reflection

In meetings, on our mats, or on our cushions, we are being invited into the same process. It is a process of integration in which we turn to face the parts of ourselves that we have disowned to learn what they have to teach us.

350.

My Zen teacher pointed out that when we disown a part of ourselves, it becomes an extremely powerful toxin that poisons our mind states, our behavior, our outcomes. Such was the case with the type of anger I learned growing up; it was the rage of someone who had disowned his sense of powerlessness. My mother's people had lived in poverty. They had faced limits in their ability to provide for their children, achieve their dreams, or live with the honor their hearts demanded. The limitations poverty imposed resulted in a crushing humiliation that was reflected back at them from every corner of their life. To be in their presence was to be in the presence of a simmering rage that would boil over into violence at the drop of a hat.

In recovery I have come to understand that my family's rage was self-protective. It was like a mad dog sitting in someone's front yard, keeping prying eyes at bay. On my cushion, I found it necessary to approach the mad dog to find out that it was protecting a house full of broken dreams. It is necessary for us to see that what we have disowned is not what it seems. My family's rage was actually disowned powerlessness, a powerlessness in the face of unremitting heartbreak. By approaching the dog, I gained access to what it was protecting. It was at this point that I could begin to forgive my own rage and the people who had taught it to me.

Reflection

An easy way to take inventory of what you have disowned is to list the people you cannot forgive. What is it about the way they are that you cannot forgive?

351.

Making a friend of difficult mind states, such as anger or jealousy, is not as hard as it sounds. Sitting quietly, doing nothing, we can either become lost in a difficult mind state, which is by definition a difficult experience, or we can recognize then accept what is happening. Acceptance allows the mind to settle. Then we have the opportunity to investigate the mind state. What is this experience that I am having? How does it feel in my body? How does it feel in my heart? What happens to my mind when it is reacting to life in this fashion? By letting go of our resistance to what is happening, we can begin to understand what is happening.

The drama of our last years of active addiction came from the tension between resisting a truth and accepting one. For most of us, our addiction had stopped being fun (if it ever was) long before we stopped using. The problem was that our first impulse was to resist. The addict crushed by the weight of addiction will resist well-meaning suggestions. Eventually it is the pain of holding on to it that makes us give up our resistance to the truth.

In meditation, we watch this same dynamic play out again and again. We watch as the mind clings to an intellectual position until it hurts so much that we let go, breathing deeply as the suffering ebbs. The next day, we hold on a little less. A few years later, we have learned to let go. When a difficult mind state arises, we can recognize the resistance within it—how resistance to the truth blocks the flow of energy, how it creates tension in the body. From recognition we soften into acceptance, allowing the energy to move. This creates the possibility of understanding. As the energy moves, we are able to see the truth for what it is.

Reflection

Before we can address a problem in our life, we must move from resistance to acceptance. Begin to feel how resistance creates tension, how acceptance creates flow.

352.

It is a subtle shift to move from resistance to recognition, from craving to acceptance, but it is decisive because we are ending our war with life on life's terms. My family learned to resist the experience of poverty, while others learned to resist racism or religious oppression. Some even learned to resist compassion for those they had enslaved. The truth was unacceptable, so they resisted. But the truth is a river. No matter how honestly we have come by our resistance, we cannot fight the river and heal at the same time.

Recovery is a healing process that is also a learning process. It could also be called a learning process that is experienced as a healing process. The person in recovery is learning how to make a choice. What we have learned so far is that to make a sound choice, we must be in conscious connection with the present moment. This connection is sustained by learning to let go into it, then resting in it. To rest in our connection to the present moment is to let go of our resistance to it. A crucial choice on the path is whether or not to let go of our resistance to life on life's terms. If we practice making this choice, we will see how concentration happens when we let go of resistance. Learning and healing happen when we can give life our undivided attention.

Reflection

Sit still and relaxed. As you breathe slowly, let go until you are entirely empty of any resistance to this moment. Notice what happens to the mind when the body is empty of resistance.

353.

Yoga allows us to ease into the experience of letting go of the fear that has driven our resistance to life on life's terms. We do not have to do it all at once, but each step is a leap of faith. Nonviolence is a leap of faith. Honesty is a leap of faith. Generosity is a leap of faith. In yoga poses we learn to let go of fear by bringing awareness into the body, noticing then releasing the extra effort we have brought to a pose or a moment. This extra effort we learn to recognize is fear. The same process takes place as we learn to sit in meditation, allowing life to hold us.

Sitting quietly, without resistance, we discover the mind's luminous nature. In conditioned reactivity the mind grabs on to thoughts, beliefs, concerns, fears, desires. In meditation we allow the mind to become open space. This intelligent space lets it all in—the insights, the connections, the understandings, the inspirations, the wisdom, the empathy, the deepest joy, the most heartfelt sorrows. This open space is our true nature. The universe, knowing this, has sent its gifts to that address.

Reflection

The universe has the job of crafting the gifts. The part we play is to be there when they arrive.

354.

To concentrate is to place our attention on one thing while forsaking all others. This has the paradoxical effect of allowing everything to come to us. When we enter recovery, we place our attention on one thing, forsaking all others. As the years go by, everything we need to create a life second to none will come to us.

My first years in recovery bore little resemblance to a traditionally successful life. I had little in terms of money, possessions, or accomplishments. I had placed my attention on something beautiful, pursuing it with a singleness of purpose. The word we used for the life I wanted was *sobriety*. This word captured something I had not even imagined existed before going to rehab. Living sober meant walking humbly and living usefully under the grace of God. This felt like an entirely decent desire to devote one's life to. It felt like outrageous good fortune to even know this desire existed, let alone to get an honest crack at living that way. So I concentrated on the most important thing, which allowed everything else to come to me.

Reflection

When working, do the most important thing. When teaching, teach the most important thing. When speaking, say the most important thing. When learning, learn the most important thing. When living, be the most important thing.

355.

The active addict has given her life to something that will never give her anything back. You could say that it gives back endless suffering, then death—but for today I want to focus on the opportunity cost of addiction. When we concentrate on one thing, we can't concentrate on something else. The addict has concentrated on something that takes but has no capacity to give. Twelve-step programs, yoga, and meditation offer a person in recovery something to be a part of that has been proven to give you more than you put into it.

A person goes to a 12-step meeting to share her experience, strength, and hope. For this investment, she receives the goodwill of all of those assembled, informed by the wisdom of countless others who have contributed to the institutional wisdom contained in 12-step programs. You walk onto a yoga mat to practice skills that have been refined over thousands of years by innumerable individuals. As you learn to apply these skills to your life, you discover the truth of who you are. As with a 12-step meeting, all you need to do to receive this gift is to show up. Meditation works the same way. We take one step toward the universe; the universe takes 10 steps toward us. All we need to do is concentrate our efforts on the path to freedom instead of the path to suffering.

Reflection

You are always on a path to somewhere, wisdom is knowing which path you are on.

Forgive

When being taught concentration, we are asked to imagine looking for a friend in a crowded room, noticing how our energy is devoted to finding the friend instead of connecting with the friend. Then we are asked to imagine looking for a friend in a room that holds only a couple of people. In this second room, we will use very little time or energy finding our friend. Instead we will be able to pour all of our energy into our actual purpose for being in the room, connection. This analogy speaks to the work we must do to eliminate distractions that would otherwise absorb our attention.

The essays in this chapter have been dedicated to both the nature of concentration and the impediments we experience as we work to bring our undivided attention to the process of recovery. My final essays will be devoted to the skill that is required to remove the last block to this superlative mind state: forgiveness. As addicts, we have judged ourselves harshly. We have judged our world harshly. This judgment lives as a constant limitation within our relationships, generating conflict even as we seek connection. To give our undivided attention to the precious lived moments of our recovery, we must be without reservation. We have lived in judgment of the living. Now is the time to forgive.

356.

When I am still, there is a period of transition in which I slowly let go of control. Allowing the body to find its natural stillness, the breath to find its natural rhythm, I rediscover the ease with which we can regain our connection to the present. As I let go into this connection, my attention is drawn to the wisdom of an open heart. There, in the midst of the wonder, rests a universe of loving-kindness. The heart is a sun that radiates wise love. As the warmth of this sun touches my pain, I experience compassion. Compassion is the knowledge that everyone is fighting a hard battle, it is the understanding that each battle is being fought by someone who is doing her best.

For a while I let go into compassion as a moment before I let go into the present. Giving compassion my undivided attention, I see a world full of space. The stories that have sealed me in now have space. The definitions that have sealed me in now have space; the history, the sorrow, the betrayal, the failures now have space. What trapped me was not so much misunderstanding as a complete lack of comprehension. Why have I lived this way? Why has this been "my best"? Why couldn't it have been better? Why couldn't I have done better, known better, loved better? The space lets in the only understanding that matters. I am not here to judge. I am here to have the courage to live with an open heart. My body remains unmoving as my spirit stands to be one with the wisdom of compassion. Standing now, my spirit has space. Through this space pours the love I was meant to bring into this world: forgiveness.

Reflection

It is probably not a coincidence that 12-step programs teach us to "let go absolutely" and the Buddha taught his students to "forgive everyone for everything." We access the wisdom of forgiveness by letting go absolutely.

357.

The recovering community humbly rebuilds. It is a group of people who are starting over again because they have no choice. What is done is done. We cannot go back. We cannot go on. We must begin again. To begin again, we must forgive ourselves, but it is too much to ask of someone who has lived as we have. We are not taking our first steps in recovery because we deserve it. We are on the path to freedom because the alternative is too much to bear.

So we learn to avoid, we learn to abandon, we allow our lives to become empty of active addiction. Emptiness has its own joy. Waking up without a hangover. Going to work without guilt. Showing up without needing anything in particular. Empty of active addiction, we begin to be full of recovery. We let people in. The people we love in recovery want the best for us. But this is not something we have wanted. We have never known what the best was or how to allow it into our lives. These new faces have new eyes that tell us there is more to us than we know. In these eyes we see someone we have never known, someone who is worthy of love, someone who is worthy of forgiveness.

Reflection

Twelve-step programs say, "Let us love you until you can love yourself." We need the eyes we look into in recovery. We will not find ourselves without them.

358.

Before I could receive compassion in the eyes of someone else, I had to be those eyes in someone else's life. It was too much to bear to simply receive compassion after a lifetime of the darkness that was the opposite of forgiveness. My 12-step program knew this; it understood the broken hearts it was meant to heal. So we were asked to pass it on by picking up chairs, making coffee, putting our hand out to newcomers. As the illness left our bodies, it became time to let the illness out of our hearts. Each small act of kindness we offered let a little of the pain out of our hearts.

After a while, I found myself driving a few young men to meetings. I had very little to give. I had a car; I could show up on time. When you were with me, you were with someone who was all in when it came to recovery. These young men are still in my life today. They are in their 50s now. They have lived a sober life. Now, when I see them, I have more to give, but they have never needed more from me than what I was able to offer so long ago. It was enough that I believed in them and the path they were choosing.

Reflection

Long before we can believe in ourselves, we can believe in each other. By coming together we are able to practice the compassion we will one day offer ourselves.

359.

When it was time for me to learn how to forgive, my teachers instructed me to begin with myself. They told me to forgive myself for being imperfect, for making mistakes, for having to learn about life by living it. This was approachable. As I practiced forgiving myself in this way, I saw how hard it was to be human, how intensely we live in the midst of uncertainty. I saw how addiction made an already difficult situation nearly impossible. I saw the difference between the person and the behavior. I saw the difference between a noun and a verb.

While the rest of the world has continued to rush toward judgment, I have learned to slow my pace. Compassion is the space for grace. I have learned to love the space. Knowing that I do not know is space. Empathy is space. Saying, "I am like that too" is grace. Lao Tzu wrote that the ancient masters were as careful as someone walking on an iced-over stream. I have learned to be as careful as someone in the presence of great pain. While the rest of the world continues to rush toward judgment, I walk carefully toward connection.

Reflection

It is not necessary to learn to forgive others. Once you have learned to forgive yourself, you have learned how to forgive everyone else.

360.

As we begin to actually forgive ourselves for being imperfect, making mistakes, and being a learner in this lifetime, we come to understand that we give the world only what we are willing to give ourselves. As we question the judgment with which we have imprisoned ourselves, we begin to question the judgment with which we have condemned the world. For a while, this can be an intellectual position, a matter of knowing that we do not know. Our judgments still have great power over us and color our view, but we have begun to question the entire process of finding fault. If we persist in the work of forgiving ourselves, there comes a moment when we feel our heart's actual intention. We move beyond an intellectual understanding into a heartfelt one.

Compassion is a spring that works its way through the meadow of our lives. While the snow is still melting, we stop using. As the first green grass begins to show, we laugh without fear. The first flowers are only buds on a branch when we know that we want our recovery to benefit all beings. The snow becomes a rushing stream as we help those who are coming along behind us. As we rest for a moment on a rock warmed by the sun, our hearts speak. "I have only ever wanted one thing, for all beings to rest in me as you are resting in this meadow."

Reflection

There is an African saying, " I am because you are." At the end of my meditation retreats, we take a moment to declare our intention that the merit of our work together be of benefit to all beings. We close the circle of our recovery when we give others the highest good we wish to experience for ourselves.

361.

Bill Wilson stood at the turning point of his life, his precarious recovery hanging in the balance as he looked into a roomful of people drinking and laughing. He could not help himself, but he knew that if he helped someone else, it would be enough. His insight was that what we give to someone else, we are giving ourselves. Twelve-step programs work because humanity is one big family. When we set time aside to listen to each other, we learn about ourselves. When we set time aside to listen to our own hearts, we come to understand the hearts all around us.

Bill Wilson said no to the idea that his destiny was somehow separate from those around him. He took the radical step of opening his heart unconditionally to another human being. Sitting in a kitchen, listening to another person share the story of his addiction, he discovered the cure for addiction: connection.

Reflection

When you listen to someone tell her story, you can feel what Bill Wilson felt.

362.

As a young person, the Buddha observed the suffering of humanity. He felt there must be something that we can do. He went into the forest to study with the Yogis. They taught him everything they knew. They taught him to find the peace of nature, to be still, to concentrate, to look inward for the answers that he was seeking. He did. Sitting quietly, resting his attention on the breath, he learned to become the forest pool welcoming all the mysterious creatures of the forest equally. Thousands of years later, people the world over still sit this way.

Once he was done, he did not believe he could teach what he had learned. Then some friends asked if he could help them. Out of compassion, he did what he could to alleviate the suffering of humanity. He sought to make his own freedom be of benefit to all beings. He taught that we are stuck in a perspective that causes us to suffer. He taught that if we wish to be free, we must let go. He taught that we must forgive everybody for everything.

Reflection

Bill Wilson and the Buddha were just human beings using the abilities every human possesses. The freedom they found was just the beginning of their journey. Their story will be yours.

363.

Unlike the life of the Buddha or Bill Wilson, little is known of the author of the Yoga Sutras. Out of the mist of history, a work of remarkable clarity emerged. It starts with a simple statement, "Now," and ends with another, "That is all." everything in between supports regaining our relationship with the present moment. For a person in recovery, the significance of these teachings cannot be overstated.

The Yoga Sutras teach a time-tested approach to healthy living, grounding physical exercises, focused breathing exercises, and a course in meditation that is second to none. I was asked recently why yoga would work for a traumatized population. I said that we certainly need to learn to meditate, but before we can do this, we must learn to feel at ease in our own skin. The Yoga Sutras create a framework for someone who has survived addiction, dealing with the effects of trauma to transform this terrible legacy into an authentic healing path. In yoga, the pain we have known becomes wisdom and compassion.

Reflection

Each of us has been given a portion of the world's pain. Yoga teaches us to take this darkness and turn it into light.

364.

There have been days when I have taken my recovery into 12-step meetings. Walking out of a fall evening into the togetherness of addicts choosing life among their peers. Taking my seat, I say a prayer of thanks. Once the meeting begins, I know myself to be in the presence of the teachings I waited all of my life to hear. There have been days when I have taken my recovery into a yoga class. Walking out of a summer afternoon into the sacred togetherness of Yogis learning freedom among their peers. Stepping onto my mat, I say a prayer of thanks. Once the class begins, I know myself to be moving through the sensations I waited all my life to process. There have been days when I have taken my recovery into a meditation hall. Walking out of a winter morning into the togetherness of Yogis learning the end of suffering among their peers. Taking my seat, I say a prayer of thanks. Resting in stillness, I know myself to be in the moment I have sought all my life.

Reflection

May our walking be of benefit to all beings.

365.

The addict in recovery is learning happiness. You do this by turning your days into moments of love and service. There are places we can go to learn how to turn our days into sacred moments. This book is a thank-you note to a few of the places that I have gone to learn happiness. I believe you will succeed. Your success will be a light in the world. This much I know. The happiness you find as you light the way for others will depend to a large extent on the company you keep. It is my hope that this book inspires you to walk into some of the rooms I have found on my path.

May you be safe

May you be healthy

May you be happy

May you be free

Acknowledgments

I would like to begin by thanking the Hay House team for their belief in this book and their unwavering support as it came together. Thank you. Words fall short when it comes to the support my wife, Mariam, has given me over the 25 years; her kindness has lit my way. Thank you. To the women and men of the 12-step community, I offer my undying gratitude. I am because you are. Thank you. To the joyous crowd of Yogis worldwide, I offer a bow and a smile; you have made a home for my heart. Thank you. To the pioneers at Spirit Rock and the Insight Meditation Society, I offer my sincerest thanks. For over a decade now I have only had to try to follow the path you are laying before me to find my way to love, joy, and meaning. Thank you. May all surfers be safe, healthy, happy, and free; you have certainly helped me to be so. Thank you. Santa Cruz's west side has made a home for my family. Whenever we have needed a friend, a soccer coach, a ride, child care, and advice on the anything and everything that make up daily life, you have been unfailingly kind. In particular you have welcomed my children in a way that has been too touching to put into words. When they have acted in a play, ran a race, and had a first day or a last one, you were there to cheer and to acknowledge the courage it takes to grow up. Thank you. There are too many names now to list, but to all of you who have been my friend, anything I have accomplished or will accomplish someday is because you were there for this healing heart. Thank you.

In closing, I will offer the world two names that are always with me. My sister, Wendy, and my dear friend Jude died of their addiction. They lived with great courage and conviction more so than I was capable of when they were alive. Their passing helped me find my courage, my conviction. I miss you every day. It is my hope that this book will give others some small sense of what it meant to look into your eyes with love. Thank you.

About the Author

Rolf Gates is one of the leading voices of modern yoga and the author of *Meditations from the Mat* and *Meditations on Intention and Being.* As a former social worker and U.S. Airborne Ranger who has practiced meditation for the last 20 years, Rolf brings his eclectic background to his practice and his teachings. His work has been featured in *Yoga Journal, Natural Health,* and *People* and as one of *Travel and Leisure*'s Top 25 Yoga Studios Around the World. He is the co-founder of the Yoga + Recovery Conference at Kripalu Center for Yoga and Health in Lenox, MA, and at Esalen Institute in Big Sur, CA, and works weekly one on one with clients in his Yoga Life Coaching program. You can visit him online at rolfgates.com.

Hay House Titles of Related Interest

YOU CAN HEAL YOUR LIFE, the movie, starring Louise Hay & Friends
(available as a 1-DVD program, an expanded 2-DVD set,
and an online streaming video)
Learn more at www.hayhouse.com/louise-movie

THE SHIFT, the movie,
starring Dr. Wayne W. Dyer
(available as a 1-DVD program, an expanded 2-DVD set,
and an online streaming video)
Learn more at www.hayhouse.com/the-shift-movie

***

HOW TO LIVE A GOOD LIFE: A Practical Guide to a Life Well Lived,
by Jonathan Fields

PERFECTLY IMPERFECT: The Art and Soul of Yoga Practice,
by Baron Baptiste

*SECRETS OF MEDITATION: A Practical Guide
to Inner Peace and Transformation,*
by davidji

*YOU HAVE 4 MINUTES TO CHANGE YOUR LIFE: Simple 4-Minute
Meditations for Inspiration, Transformation, and True Bliss,*
by Rebekah Borucki

All of the above are available at your local bookstore,
or may be ordered by contacting Hay House (see next page).

***

We hope you enjoyed this Hay House book. If you'd like to receive our online catalog featuring additional information on Hay House books and products, or if you'd like to find out more about the Hay Foundation, please contact:

Hay House, Inc., P.O. Box 5100, Carlsbad, CA 92018-5100
(760) 431-7695 or (800) 654-5126
(760) 431-6948 (fax) or (800) 650-5115 (fax)
www.hayhouse.com® • www.hayfoundation.org

———

Published in Australia by:
Hay House Australia Pty. Ltd., 18/36 Ralph St., Alexandria NSW 2015
Phone: 612-9669-4299 • *Fax:* 612-9669-4144 • www.hayhouse.com.au

Published in the United Kingdom by:
Hay House UK, Ltd., Astley House, 33 Notting Hill Gate, London W11 3JQ
Phone: 44-20-3675-2450 • *Fax:* 44-20-3675-2451 • www.hayhouse.co.uk

Published in India by: Hay House Publishers India,
Muskaan Complex, Plot No. 3, B-2, Vasant Kunj, New Delhi 110 070
Phone: 91-11-4176-1620 • *Fax:* 91-11-4176-1630 • www.hayhouse.co.in

———

Access New Knowledge.
Anytime. Anywhere.

Learn and evolve at your own pace
with the world's leading experts.

www.hayhouseU.com

Free e-newsletters
from Hay House, the Ultimate
Resource for Inspiration

Be the first to know about Hay House's free downloads, special offers, giveaways, contests, and more!

 Get exclusive excerpts from our latest releases and videos from *Hay House Present Moments*.

 Our *Digital Products Newsletter* is the perfect way to stay up-to-date on our latest discounted eBooks, featured mobile apps, and Live Online and On Demand events.

 Learn with real benefits! *HayHouseU.com* is your source for the most innovative online courses from the world's leading personal growth experts. Be the first to know about new online courses and to receive exclusive discounts.

 Enjoy uplifting personal stories, how-to articles, and healing advice, along with videos and empowering quotes, within *Heal Your Life*.

 Have an inspirational story to tell and a passion for writing? Sharpen your writing skills with insider tips from *Your Writing Life*.

Sign Up Now!

Get inspired, educate yourself, get a complimentary gift, and share the wisdom!

Visit www.hayhouse.com/newsletters to sign up today!

HAY HOUSE

HAYHOUSE RADIO
radio for your soul®

HAYHOUSE
online learning

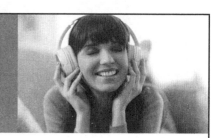

Hay House Podcasts
Bring Fresh, Free Inspiration Each Week!

Hay House proudly offers a selection of life-changing audio content via our most popular podcasts!

Hay House Meditations Podcast

Features your favorite Hay House authors guiding you through meditations designed to help you relax and rejuvenate. Take their words into your soul and cruise through the week!

Dr. Wayne W. Dyer Podcast

Discover the timeless wisdom of Dr. Wayne W. Dyer, world-renowned spiritual teacher and affectionately known as "the father of motivation." Each week brings some of the best selections from the 10-year span of Dr. Dyer's talk show on HayHouseRadio.com.

Hay House World Summit Podcast

Over 1 million people from 217 countries and territories participate in the massive online event known as the Hay House World Summit. This podcast offers weekly mini-lessons from World Summits past as a taste of what you can hear during the annual event, which occurs each May.

Hay House Radio Podcast

Listen to some of the best moments from HayHouseRadio.com, featuring expert authors such as Dr. Christiane Northrup, Anthony William, Caroline Myss, James Van Praagh, and Doreen Virtue discussing topics such as health, self-healing, motivation, spirituality, positive psychology, and personal development.

Hay House Live Podcast

Enjoy a selection of insightful and inspiring lectures from Hay House Live, an exciting event series that features Hay House authors and leading experts in the fields of alternative health, nutrition, intuitive medicine, success, and more! Feel the electricity of our authors engaging with a live audience, and get motivated to live your best life possible!

Find Hay House podcasts on iTunes, or visit
www.HayHouse.com/podcasts for more info.

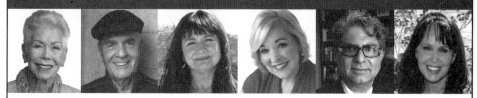